DASH
for Weight Loss

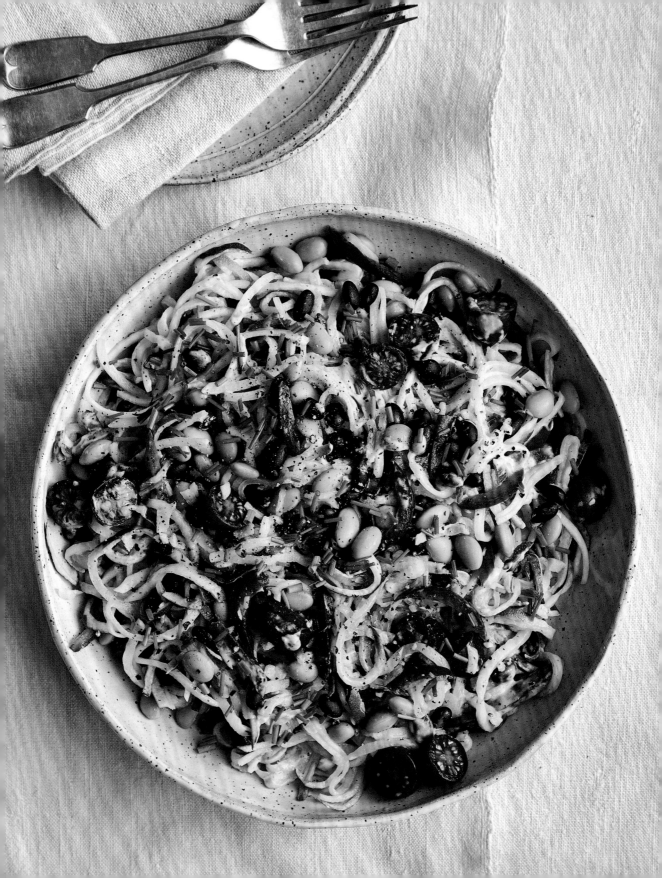

DASH
for Weight Loss

An Easy-to-Follow Plan for
Losing Weight, Increasing Energy,
and Lowering Blood Pressure

Jennifer Koslo
PhD, RDN, LDN, CPT

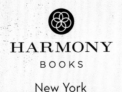

HARMONY
BOOKS

New York

To my parents, Erma and Walter, for their continued support
of all of my endeavors.

Published in the United States by Harmony Books, an imprint
of Random House, a division of Penguin Random House LLC,
New York.

Harmony Books is a registered trademark, and the Circle colo-
phon is a trademark of Penguin Random House LLC.

Library of Congress Cataloging-in-Publication Data
has been applied for.

ISBN 978-1-9848-2487-5
Ebook ISBN 978-1-9848-2488-2

Printed in China

Book design by Nick Caruso Design
Photographs by Hélène Dujardin
Cover design by Nick Caruso Design
Cover photograph by Hélène Dujardin

10 9 8 7 6 5 4 3

First Edition

Contents

Introduction

If you're trying to improve your heart health, lower your blood pressure, lose weight, and boost your metabolism, it's time to ditch the latest fad diet. You can accomplish all of these goals and still fill your plate with delicious, wholesome foods without feeling deprived by following the DASH (Dietary Approaches to Stop Hypertension) diet.

The DASH diet was specifically developed to help people lower high blood pressure (hypertension), and is promoted by the National Heart, Lung, and Blood Institute (NHLBI), which is part of the National Institutes of Health.[1] Rooted in proven science, DASH has been consistently ranked by *U.S. News & World Report* as the "best overall" diet.

The DASH eating plan encourages you to reduce the amount of sodium in your diet while increasing your daily servings of nutrient-rich foods, specifically focusing on three key minerals that can help lower blood pressure: calcium, magnesium, and potassium.

In as little as two weeks, you may be able to lower your blood pressure by several points. Over time, following DASH can significantly reduce your health risks, and simultaneously help you to shed unwanted pounds.

Although the DASH diet was not designed with weight loss as a primary goal, the NHLBI recognizes it as an amazing side effect. They've created a range of plans that provide from 1,200 to 3,100 calories per day, so you can choose one that works best for your dietary needs. Each plan consists of a recommended number of food group servings so you can follow a targeted weight-loss plan that ensures nutrient needs are met. DASH is full of variety, and easy to follow as a sustainable, lifelong dietary choice. Choosing DASH as your eating plan can kick-start your new healthy routine as DASH is not a fad diet but rather is based on those tried-and-true concepts that are essential to planning a healthy diet.

The NHLBI website provides a wealth of information about DASH, including tips for starting and following the diet. Among the Internet, books, and cookbooks, there is no shortage of information on the DASH diet; however, this book is distinctive. As a registered dietitian nutritionist (RDN) and personal trainer certified by the American Council on Exercise, I have worked with numerous clients on weight-loss regimens, wellness protocols, exercise programming, and chronic disease prevention. As a result of my work, I have developed a wide-ranging knowledge of food and nutrition that complements my love of cooking

and recipe development. Throughout my career, I've worked extensively with the DASH diet, and my professional expertise has inspired me to create this all-in-one guidebook to help you reduce your risks for chronic disease. You'll also get fit and lose weight as you enjoy filling and delicious foods.

This book consists of three parts. The first covers all the basics: health benefits, the science behind the DASH diet, strategies for making a long-term lifestyle change, and the basics of weight management. The second teaches you how to set yourself up for success by making your kitchen DASH-friendly and learning how to become a meal planning, shopping, prepping, and cooking pro. It also includes a meal plan and exercise plan, where I pull it all together with four weeks of DASH menus and physical activity schedules. And the third shares tasty recipes for all kinds of meals, snacks, sauces, sides, and desserts.

Get ready to fill your pantry with whole grains, vegetables, fruits, low-fat dairy products, fish, poultry, beans, nuts, and oil. Prepare to cut back on processed foods, trans fats, red meat, and excess sodium and sugar. Invite your family to join you. Some adjustments will be small, but the results can be significant. You have already taken an important first step by reading this book and I am honored to be your guide to becoming a healthier, lighter you!

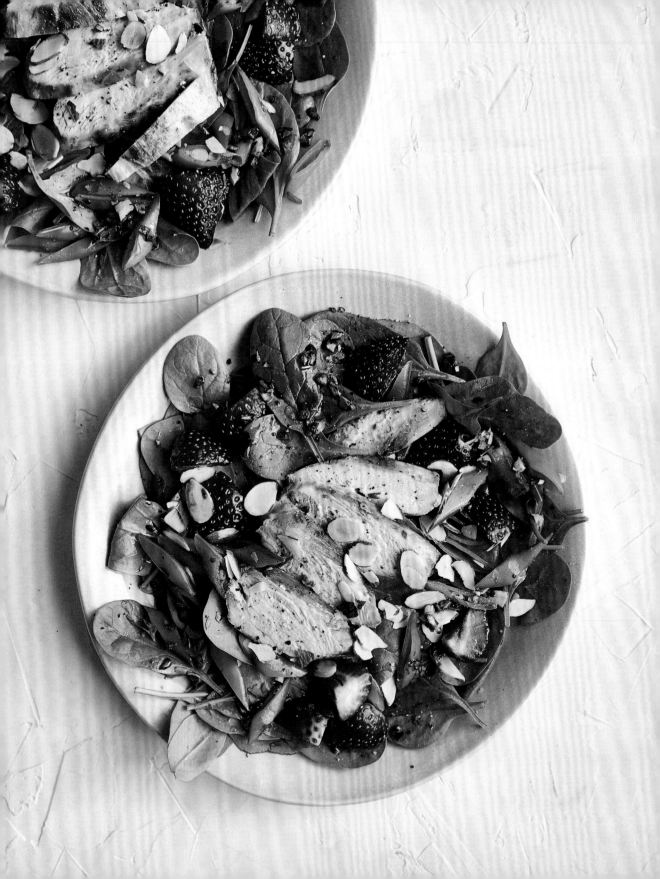

DASH: HOW THE HEALTHIEST DIET WORKS

Health Benefits of DASH

The DASH diet has helped people with hypertension and pre-hypertension lower their blood pressure for over twenty years. By reducing blood pressure, this diet can also decrease the need for costly medications. Even if hypertension is not your main concern, DASH is a great option for anyone who wants to adopt a healthy diet in general. Because DASH emphasizes moderate portions and whole, unprocessed foods, a beneficial "side effect" for most people is weight loss.

DASH is actually quite simple. It encourages you to eat less of the foods you already know really aren't the best options for your waistline or health, including fast food, processed foods, refined carbohydrates, red meat, sugar-filled beverages, prepackaged dishes, and salty foods—you get the idea. And it includes a variety of foods to eat *more* of, such as whole grains, vegetables, fruits, beans, nuts, healthy fats, lean meats, and low-fat dairy.

DASH is not a low-carb diet. It is not a vegan or vegetarian diet, or even one that is restrictively low in sodium. The original DASH trial included a sodium level of 2,300 milligrams per day, which is the amount recommended in the 2015–2020 Dietary Guidelines for Americans. Yet, after only two weeks of following the DASH diet, the participants in the study experienced a drop in blood pressure.[1]

In addition to lower blood pressure, some of the other benefits to following the DASH diet include:

- Lower cholesterol
- A reduced risk of certain chronic diseases
- Improved control of type 2 diabetes
- Weight loss
- Better overall nutrition

However, keep in mind that the amount of time it takes to lower your blood pressure depends on a variety of factors including your age, gender, current health status, race, weight, co-morbidities (for example, type 2 diabetes, kidney disease), and so on. Please do not stop taking your medications (high blood pressure, diabetes, or any other pre-scription medication) when you embark on the DASH diet, as this could put you at risk for life-threatening complications. Always consult with your physician and let him/her know you are making dietary and lifestyle changes so that they may adjust your medications accordingly when the time is right.

Additionally, it is very important to have realistic expectations of outcomes from following the DASH diet. The older we get, the harder it becomes to lose weight due to a slower metabolism and loss of muscle mass. In other words, what worked for weight loss at age 20 won't work at 30, 40, or 50+. But you can still make significant changes in your health—just be patient. Focus on progress rather than perfection. View it as a lifestyle change and not a temporary fix. Even if you don't notice immediate changes in your weight, within two to four weeks, you should notice improvements in your digestion, concentration, energy level, and body shape.

Hypertension Basics

You have probably heard the saying that high blood pressure is a "silent killer," but what exactly does that mean? High blood pressure (hypertension) often has no obvious symptoms, and if left undiagnosed and untreated, the damage it does to your circulatory system could increase your risk for a heart attack or stroke, and can lead to heart disease, kidney disease, heart failure, and damage to your eyes.[2]

While everyone wants to have a healthy blood pressure, the parameters for what

DOES DIETARY CHOLESTEROL STILL MATTER?

Nutrition guidelines can certainly be confusing. For years, the public was told to limit dietary cholesterol to no more than 240 milligrams per day. Now with the 2015–2020 Dietary Guidelines for Americans, the limit on cholesterol has been completely removed. So what gives? The cholesterol in our blood does not come directly from cholesterol in the foods we eat. With that said, what we eat can still raise our blood cholesterol. The type and amount of *fat* we eat is what makes the impact on our cholesterol, and some fats are more harmful than others. The worst type of fat for your heart and cholesterol is trans fats, which the Food and Drug Administration has determined to be unsafe and therefore removed from our food supply. This change officially went into effect on June 21, 2018, so you should look for 0 grams of trans fats on ingredient labels or in foods. Saturated fats, such as those found in animal products, also raise "bad" or LDL cholesterol; however, recent research suggests that some types, such as the fats found in chocolate and coconut oil, do so less than others.

Bottom line: Avoid trans fats all together and keep saturated fats and tropical oils in check. Choose extra-virgin olive oil most often.

Know Your Numbers: Blood Pressure Readings Explained

The chart below shows the newly defined categories. If you have your numbers, you can see what they mean.

BLOOD PRESSURE CATEGORY	SYSTOLIC MM HG (UPPER NUMBER)	AND/OR	DIASTOLIC MM HG (LOWER NUMBER)
NORMAL	Less than 120	and	Less than 80
ELEVATED	120 to 129	and	Less than 80
HIGH BLOOD PRESSURE STAGE 1	130 to 139	or	80 to 89
HIGH BLOOD PRESSURE STAGE 2	140 or higher	or	90 or higher
HYPERTENSIVE CRISIS (CONSULT YOUR DOCTOR IMMEDIATELY)	Higher than 180	and/or	Higher than 120

(Source: American Heart Association, 2018)

FULL-FAT, LOW-FAT, OR FAT-FREE DAIRY?

DASH has been tested using full-fat dairy products instead of low-fat or fat-free to see if adding certain foods will keep it as beneficial. In a recent study published in the *American Journal of Clinical Nutrition,* researchers found that the DASH diet with higher-fat dairy was just as beneficial in lowering blood pressure as the standard DASH diet.[3] To compensate for the extra calories, participants consumed less sugar. The takeaway here is that it is possible to accommodate a variety of preferences when following DASH and still obtain significant health benefits.

qualifies as "normal" or "healthy" just got a lot stricter based on new guidelines released at the end of 2017 by a joint committee of the American College of Cardiology and the American Heart Association.[4]

Blood pressure readings are expressed in millimeters of mercury—the unit is abbreviated as "mm Hg." The new blood pressure guidelines categorize hypertension as a reading of 130/80 mm Hg from the previous standard of 140/90 mm Hg.[5] This change increased the percentage of US adults with high blood pressure from 32 percent to 46 percent—almost half of all Americans. Use the chart on page 11 to see what your blood pressure readings indicate.

In order to understand your readings, it is helpful to know how your blood pressure works, without getting too scientific. *Blood pressure* is the force that your heart exerts against the resistance that your arteries create to keep blood flowing through your body. When you get your blood pressure taken, it's expressed as a measurement with two numbers: For example: 120/80 mm Hg. The top number (*systolic*) refers to the amount of pressure in your arteries during the contraction of your heart muscle. The bottom number (*diastolic*) refers to your blood pressure when your heart muscle is in between beats. Both numbers are important for determining if your heart is working too hard to pump blood to the rest of your body.

Risk Factors

There are a number of factors that can increase your risk of high blood pressure that are simply out of your control. These include being over age 50, being male or a postmenopausal female, being black, and/or having a family history of high blood pressure.

Preventive Measures

On the flip side, there are many preventive steps you can take to lower your risk of developing high blood pressure that are *entirely* within your control. These include:

- MAINTAINING A HEALTHY WEIGHT
  Almost two-thirds of the people suffering from obesity are at risk for high blood pressure. If you are overweight, losing

just 5 percent of your body weight or 5 to 10 pounds can make a positive impact on your blood pressure readings.

- **FOLLOWING THE DASH DIET** The DASH diet can lower your blood pressure and your cholesterol, which if elevated can increase the risk of suffering complications from hypertension.

- **REDUCING YOUR SODIUM INTAKE** Too much sodium in your diet can cause your body to retain fluid and also causes your arteries to constrict, both of which raise blood pressure.

- **INCREASING YOUR POTASSIUM INTAKE** Potassium helps balance the sodium in your cells and causes the cells

in your arteries to relax, which lowers blood pressure.

- **GETTING ACTIVE** Aim to be active every day and meet the minimum recommended 150 minutes of moderate cardiovascular exercise per week (exercise will be discussed in-depth later).

- **MANAGING YOUR STRESS** Chronic stress can elevate your blood pressure. Take steps to incorporate daily relaxation and meditation techniques.

- **LIMITING YOUR ALCOHOL INTAKE** Long-term heavy drinking may cause damage to your heart, but more directly, having several drinks within a short period of time can temporarily raise your blood pressure. Moderate drinking is defined as two drinks per day for men, and one drink per day for women. One drink is equal to one 12-ounce beer with 5 percent alcohol, or one 5-ounce glass of wine, or 1½ ounces of 80-proof liquor.

- **TAKING STEPS TO STOP SMOKING IF YOU SMOKE** Nicotine raises blood pressure. Smoking is also a risk factor for coronary artery disease and stroke.

- **TAKING STEPS TO MANAGE OTHER HEALTH CONDITIONS** Certain chronic conditions including diabetes, sleep apnea, thyroid problems, and kidney disease increase your blood pressure, so talk with your physician to ensure you are doing everything you can to control your risk factors.

- **MANAGING MEDICATIONS** There are many different classes of medications used to treat hypertension. By following the

EATING OUT ON THE DASH DIET

- Ask how the foods are prepared and choose simple meals: e.g., grilled chicken or fish with steamed vegetables, salads with dressing on the side, broth-based soups, baked potato with toppings on the side.

- Choose water for your drink of choice.

- Choose baked or grilled options and ask servers to have the kitchen prepare your food with little oil/butter.

- Avoid foods that typically contain a lot of added fat and sodium including tuna, chicken, and egg salads; taco bowls, and menu items with creamy sauces like Alfredo.

DASH diet you may be able to reduce your need for drugs. Do not stop or change your dosage without your physicians' advice.

Dietary Patterns

Research carried out before the launch of the original DASH study showed that *eating patterns* (as opposed to single nutrients) can affect blood pressure in people with moderate to severe hypertension. In the early 1990s, due to the increasing and troubling prevalence of high blood pressure in the US, the National Institutes of Health (NIH) proposed funding to further research the role of dietary patterns on blood pressure—thus DASH was born. The Dietary Approaches to Stop Hypertension diet was developed and used in a large study, which began in 1993 and ended in 1997.[6]

The DASH experimental diet included higher levels of nutrients known to be associated with low blood pressure including the minerals potassium, magnesium, and calcium, as well as dietary fiber and higher levels of antioxidants. The diet did not restrict sodium levels, which were kept to an average of 3,000 milligrams (mg) per day (more than the recommended 2,300 mg per day).

Simply put, DASH includes more servings of vegetables, fruits, whole grains, low-fat and fat-free dairy products, nuts, and legumes. DASH contains smaller amounts of red meats and saturated fats. This eating pattern translates into a daily diet very rich in calcium, magnesium, potassium, and fiber, and low in saturated fats. After just two weeks following the DASH diet, participants lowered both their systolic and diastolic blood pressure significantly.

Many trials have been conducted since that first landmark DASH study, including those with and without sodium restriction. Scientists have compiled the results of these many studies and have found on average that people reduce their systolic blood pressure by 6.7 mm Hg and their diastolic blood pressure by 3.5 mm Hg in just two weeks. When sodium is kept to 1,500 mg per day, the results are even better.

The higher amounts of potassium, magnesium, calcium, and fiber plus lower amounts of sodium and saturated fat in the DASH diet improve the electrolyte balance in the body, allowing it to excrete excess fluid, which contributes to high blood pressure. These nutrients also promote relaxation of the blood vessels, which in turn reduces blood pressure. Additionally, because the diets of many Americans are lacking in these nutrients, following the principles of DASH can correct those deficiencies and help people feel better.

DASH Guidelines

Today, two versions of the DASH guidelines are promoted. You can choose the one that is right for you depending on your health needs:

- STANDARD DASH DIET limits sodium consumption to 2,300 mg per day (the amount recommended by the 2015–2020 Dietary Guidelines for Americans).

- LOWER-SODIUM DASH DIET limits sodium consumption to 1,500 mg per day.

10 EASY WAYS TO TRANSITION TO THE DASH DIET FOR WEIGHT LOSS

1. Incorporate two to three meatless meals per week: Start a new tradition by incorporating "meatless Mondays" into your weekly routine. Enjoying more plant-based meals is good for your heart, your waistline, and the environment.

2. Start your meals with a fresh green salad: You can knock out 3+ servings of vegetables by starting one of your meals with a nutrient-rich salad. Try 2 cups of baby kale with tomatoes, mushrooms, and carrots plus a drizzle of extra-virgin olive oil.

3. Fill half of your plate at lunch and dinner with vegetables: Filling half of your plate with nonstarchy vegetables at lunch and dinner will boost your intake of vitamins, minerals, and fiber and keep you from feeling deprived.

4. DASH-ify your snacks: Aim for snacks that include a balance of nutrients to keep you full and help meet your daily food servings. Try Greek yogurt with berries and almonds, or a string cheese with an apple in place of processed snacks.

5. Swap soda for fat-free or low-fat milk (or fortified plant-based milk): Soda is just empty calories. It's much better for your body to replace it with a calcium-rich drink, or simply switch to water.

6. Swap one of your daily servings of starchy carbs for beans or legumes: If you normally have bread and a grain with dinner, replace one of those with ½ cup of beans or legumes. This will add key minerals, protein, and fiber to your diet.

7. Be conscious of your sodium intake: You need some sodium in your diet and the standard DASH diet allows up to 2,300 mg. Don't go overboard by cutting out all salt, but do be conscious of how much you are consuming each day.

8. Replace unhealthy fats with healthy fats: Avocado makes a nutritious replacement for butter on bread; pureed prunes and applesauce are terrific oil replacements in muffins, pancakes, and quick breads like banana bread; make extra-virgin olive oil your oil of choice.

9. Become a label-reading pro: Start checking the nutrition facts panel. Choose foods low in sodium and saturated fats and high in fiber.

10. Carve out time and space in your schedule for meal planning, shopping, prepping, and cooking: Make it a habit to set aside time one or two days each week to plan your meals and do some prep work. Sunday afternoons are a great time for this.

Balanced Eating Plan That Works

One of the biggest reasons for the success of DASH is that it includes a wide variety of foods with ample serving sizes, and it doesn't eliminate food groups. DASH is more about *adding* nutrient-dense foods to your diet, and slightly restricting the more harmful foods and nutrients.

Even more important, you don't have to get hung up on meeting specific goals on a per-meal basis or even a per-day basis. Rather, DASH focuses on the sum total of your dietary pattern over the course of several days or a week—something I'll show you how to monitor easily with some basic meal-planning tips.

Always think in terms of what you can *add* to your meals to make them more "DASH-like." Focus on making your diet a little better each day, rather than aiming for a "perfect" diet that ends up being counter-productive for long-term success.

Key Minerals to Lower Blood Pressure

The secret to the blood-pressure-lowering effects of the DASH diet is its emphasis on a dietary pattern high in three key minerals: calcium, magnesium, and potassium.

WHAT EACH MINERAL DOES	RECOMMENDED AMOUNT (USDA)				
	FEMALE 19 to 50 years	FEMALE 50+ years	MALE 19 to 50 years	MALE 50+years	DASH (2,000-calorie diet)
CALCIUM: Helps regulate blood pressure by tightening and relaxing blood vessels as needed **Good sources:** Dairy products, fortified plant milks, fortified orange juice, tofu, turnip greens, kale, bok choy, broccoli	1,000 mg	1,200 mg	1,000 mg	1,000 mg	1,250 mg
MAGNESIUM: Helps regulate hundreds of body systems including blood pressure, blood sugar, and muscle and nerve function **Good sources:** Almonds, spinach, cashews, peanuts, black beans, whole-wheat bread, edamame, avocado, brown rice, potatoes	310 to 320 mg	320 mg	400 to 420 mg	420 mg	500 mg
POTASSIUM: Important for muscle function including relaxing the walls of the blood vessels, which lowers blood pressure; normal levels are important for the conduction of electrical signals in the heart **Good sources:** Apricots, lentils, prunes, winter squash, raisins, potatoes, kidney beans, orange juice, banana, milk, spinach	2,600 mg	2,600 mg	3,400 mg	3,400 mg	4,700 mg

Recommended Daily Servings

The DASH diet doesn't list specific foods to eat. Instead, it recommends a dietary pattern that focuses on the number of servings of different food groups. The following table lists the recommended daily servings (except where weekly is noted) for three different calorie levels.[7]

FOOD GROUP	1,600 CALORIES	1,800 CALORIES	2,000 CALORIES
Grains	6	6	6 to 8
Vegetables	3 to 4	4 to 5	4 to 5
Fruits	4	4 to 5	4 to 5
Fat-free or low-fat dairy products	2 to 3	2 to 3	2 to 3
Lean meats, poultry, and fish	3 to 4 or less	6 or less	6 or less
Nuts, seeds, and legumes	3 to 4 per week	4 per week	4 to 5 per week
Fats and oils	2	2 to 3	2 to 3
Sweets and added sugars	3 or less per week	5 or less per week	5 or less per week
Maximum sodium per day	2,300 mg	2,300 mg	2,300 mg

DASH Foods

DASH doesn't specify exact foods to eat; instead it recommends including *more* nutrient-dense foods and *fewer* foods that studies have shown contribute to high blood pressure.

ENJOY FREELY	ENJOY IN MODERATION	ENJOY OCCASIONALLY	EAT LESS	AVOID
• Vegetables • Fruits • Low-fat or fat-free dairy • Legumes (lentils, beans, and peas)	• Whole grains • Nuts, seeds • Fish • Lean poultry • Eggs	• Lean red meat • Full-fat diary	• Fatty meats • Sugar, sweets • Processed foods • Sodium/salt • Saturated fats	• Trans fats • Cured and processed meats

Serving Sizes and Nutrients of Note

If you are confused about what a serving size is, then you are not alone. Typically, we think in terms of portion sizes, yet portion sizes can be one or two servings depending on the food. The following table lists standard serving sizes, examples, and the nutrients of note for each food group.

FOOD GROUP	SERVING SIZES	NUTRIENTS OF NOTE
Grains: Look for whole grains (whole-wheat pasta, brown rice, quinoa) and try to avoid processed grains (regular pasta and white bread) as whole grains have more nutrients and fiber.	1 slice bread 1 ounce dry cereal ½ cup cooked rice, pasta, or hot cereal	Significant source of energy, B vitamins, minerals, and fiber
Vegetables: Choose fresh or frozen or no-salt-added canned.	1 cup raw leafy vegetable ½ cup cut-up raw or cooked vegetable ½ cup vegetable juice	Rich sources of potassium, magnesium, and fiber, and many vitamins
Fruits: Choose fresh or frozen or no-sugar-added canned.	1 medium piece fruit ¼ cup dried fruit ½ cup fresh, frozen, or canned fruit ½ cup 100% fruit juice	Rich sources of potassium, magnesium, and fiber, and many vitamins
Fat-free or 1% low-fat dairy products	1 cup milk or yogurt 1½ ounces cheese	Significant sources of protein, vitamin D, and calcium
Lean meats, poultry, and fish	1 ounce cooked meat, poultry, or fish 1 egg	Rich sources of protein, iron, zinc, B vitamins, and magnesium
Nuts, seeds, and legumes	⅓ cup or 1½ ounces nuts 2 tablespoons peanut butter 2 tablespoons or ½ ounce seeds ½ cup cooked legumes (lentils, beans, or peas)	Significant sources of energy, magnesium, protein, potassium, and fiber
Fats and oils	1 teaspoon soft margarine 1 teaspoon vegetable oil 1 tablespoon mayonnaise 2 tablespoons salad dressing	DASH recommends a goal of 27% total calories from fat, 6% or less from saturated fat
Sweets and added sugars	1 tablespoon sugar 1 tablespoon jelly or jam ½ cup sorbet	Sweets should be low in fat

Losing Weight with DASH

One 2010 study published in the *Archives of Internal Medicine* found that overweight followers of DASH who also exercised lost an average of 19 pounds over four months.[8] In the next chapter you'll learn how to lose weight by following DASH and exercising. The meal plans I present later are designed for a 1,600-calorie diet with tips for increasing the calorie level depending on your needs and level of activity. Because DASH is so rich in servings of high-volume, low-calorie, high-fiber foods, you can easily sustain this eating pattern for the long haul without feeling deprived and meet your weight-loss goals. Below is an example of what you might eat in a typical day following a 1,600-calorie DASH diet:

- BREAKFAST ¼ cup dry steel-cut oatmeal cooked in 1 cup fat-free milk, 2 tablespoons chopped walnuts, ½ banana

- MORNING SNACK Medium apple with ½ tablespoon almond butter

- LUNCH 3 ounces cooked chicken breast, ½ cup brown rice, 1 cup steamed zucchini, 2 cups baby spinach with ¼ cup avocado slices

- AFTERNOON SNACK 2 tablespoons hummus with 10 baby carrots

- DINNER ½ cup black beans, 4 ounces grilled salmon, 1 small sweet potato, 1 cup steamed broccoli, 2 cups baby spring mix with 2 teaspoons extra-virgin olive oil

- EVENING SNACK ½ cup low-fat (2%) Greek yogurt with 1 cup raspberries

- NUTRITIONAL ANALYSIS Calories: 1,600; Total fat: 49 g; Saturated fat: 8 g; Cholesterol: 160 mg; Sodium: 921 mg; Potassium: 3,248 mg; Total carbohydrates 196 g; Fiber: 49 g; Sugars: 54 g; Protein: 107 g

Making DASH Work for You

DASH is suitable for ages 2 on up and can reduce the risk for developing chronic diseases at any age. Involve your whole family in transitioning to DASH, and make planning meals and cooking a family affair. It's never too early to start your children on the path to good health.

The recipes in this book are meant to appeal to both young and old, are quick to prepare, and definitely delicious. If you have other health conditions such as celiac, you can find gluten-free options provided in the recipes as well. And while DASH is not a vegetarian diet, it can easily become one with its emphasis on plant proteins, vegetables, whole grains, nuts, and seeds.

Even if you are a vegan, DASH can still work for you. Many of the recipes in this book are "accidentally" vegan, and where appropriate I've given tips to modify others to make them vegan. If you are concerned that following DASH will take too much time or work or cost too much, don't be. I will give you time-saving tips, budget-saving tips, and ways to cut down on food waste. Wherever you are starting, you can make DASH work for you. The potential in terms of health and longevity will be well worth it.

Essentials of Weight Loss

One of the biggest struggles people have with losing weight is simply getting started. The next is choosing from the overwhelming number of options telling you what to eat, what not to eat, and when and how to exercise. And while many of those options will help you lose weight in the short term, the bulk of diets circulating in the media use extreme measures, are not based on science, and will leave you less healthy, underfueled, grumpy, and unsatisfied. Make no mistake: For the majority of people, losing weight is not easy. It takes time, commitment, and hard work, and is full of ups and downs.

On top of that, most people approach weight loss through short-term solutions—a quick-fix diet or cleanse full of restriction, deprivation, and isolation made bearable only by the sheer fact that it is short-term. But there has to be another, more sane and balanced, approach, doesn't there? Gearing up to follow the DASH eating plan for weight loss should get you excited because the focus is on *adding* a bounty of fresh, nutritious foods that will boost your energy and feed your cravings, while crowding out the foods that leave you feeling fatigued, hungry, and unsatisfied.

In this chapter, you'll learn how to use key weight-loss and behavior-change strategies in conjunction with the DASH eating plan for lasting weight loss. You will also be tasked with finding your "why" to commit to becoming a healthier, fitter person. I will explain the basics of weight management and metabolism, provide behavior modification tips and tricks you can start using today, include lists of healthy snacks and other key components essential to weight-loss success, and discuss ways to boost your activity. By following the plan outlined in this book, you will have the information and tools you need to make positive changes to your eating habits, and engage in a balanced program of physical activity so that weight loss should follow as a natural and welcome effect.

Weight Management Basics

Common sense and conventional weight-loss theories have long supported the notion that weight management (maintaining the same weight) boils down to a simple math equation where calories in should equal calories out. One pound of fat equals 3,500 calories, and to lose one pound per week, a deficit of 3,500 calories needs to be made over the course of seven days, or about 500 calories less per day. The most effective approach to this is through a combination of diet and exercise: Eat 250 calories less and do purposeful, physical activity that burns 250 calories. In other words, eat less, move more. Pretty simple, right? Then why doesn't this always work?

Researchers now know that there are many factors in addition to diet and activity that affect your weight and can make losing those extra pounds excruciatingly slow. Some of these include slowed metabolism, lack of sleep, too much stress, environmental toxins, side effects of certain medications, hormonal status (i.e., menopause), low calcium status, and gut bacteria that are out of balance. So the first thing to do is stop beating yourself up if you have not succeeded at lasting weight loss. You are not lazy. Everything from our biology to our toxic food environment to our emotions makes weight loss an uphill battle. The good news is that you can take steps to overcome some of these obstacles. Here are some simple strategies to get you started on supercharging your weight loss:

- **CHANGE YOUR PERSPECTIVE** If your only motivation to lose weight is to look a certain way, it will be hard to lose weight permanently. A key to lasting weight loss is finding your "*whys*"—those reasons that will motivate you on days when you feel like throwing in the towel. Take some time to get clear on your "whys" and write down at least three. Consider concrete objectives such as: to lower your risk factors for type 2 diabetes, to have more energy to play with your kids, to have more energy so you can take the stairs instead of the elevator, to sleep better, so you can take that hiking trip you have wanted to. These are just a few. It is critical that you actually take the time to do this.

- **TAKE STOCK OF YOUR LIFESTYLE** If you want a healthy lifestyle, then you need to take stock of a few things and consider making changes where needed to increase your chances of success. For example, are you willing to get up 30 minutes earlier so you have time to take a walk, eat a healthy breakfast, and pack a lunch for work? You might have to start by keeping a 24-hour time diary—if you have never done this, you will be amazed at how insightful they are! How much time do you spend on your phone? Watching TV? Once you have an idea of how you spend your time, you can use all of those snippets and pockets of unproductive time for scheduling meal planning, cooking, exercising, practicing self-care, sleeping, and so on.

- **KNOW YOUR HEALTH RISKS** Body mass index and waist circumference are two screening tools you can use to assess your health risks for chronic disease. Body mass index (BMI) is a measure of height and weight (weight in kilograms divided by the square of height in meters), and a high BMI can be an indicator of high body fat. Keep in mind that BMI is not accurate for athletic individuals and it is not diagnostic of your health. However, it is a good general screening tool. Waist circumference is another screening tool you can use. A waist circumference of 40 inches or more in men or 35 inches or more in women is associated with health problems such as type 2 diabetes, heart disease, and high blood pressure. The National Heart, Lung, and Blood Institute has an online calculator you can use to quickly find your BMI. It can be found at https://www.nhlbi.nih.gov/health/educational/lose_wt/BMI/bmicalc.htm.

- **IMPROVE YOUR SLEEP** Most of us know that when we lose sleep, we are often too tired to exercise and make less healthful food choices. Keeping a consistent sleeping schedule, setting up a pleasant sleeping environment, and making sure electronics stay out of the bedroom can go a long way toward improving sleep. It also may help to practice relaxation techniques, to refrain from eating close to bedtime, and to make sure you get plenty of sunshine and physical activity during the day.

- **TRACK YOUR CALORIES FOR A DAY OR TWO** Think of the calories you eat and spend like your money: You probably know how much money you make and how much you spend, even if only by the balance in your checking account. With calories and weight loss, before you set your goals and create your road map, you need to have a good idea of what you are doing now. Tracking calories is onerous for most people, so this is just a short-term exercise to increase your weight-loss success. Choose from one of the thousands of free apps or online programs, or even keep track by hand. Find out how many calories you eat in a typical day or two. Keep this information handy for goal setting and when you start using the meal plans.

- **GET A GENERAL IDEA OF HOW MANY CALORIES YOU NEED** Assuming you tracked your calories, the next thing you need to do is determine how many calories you need per day. This can be tricky because of the many factors that influence this number including age, level of activity, co-morbidities like type 2 diabetes, medications, and so on. As you go through this activity, keep in mind that calculations are a "best guess estimate." If you really want to zero in on your calorie needs, then you can have your Resting Metabolic Rate (RMR) measured. If you are interested in having your RMR measured, check your area for local sports medicine clinics, health clubs, and doctor's offices for availability of this service. However, if you can't do that, formulas are a great place to start. The easiest thing to do would be to use an online calculator but if you want to do it yourself, the math is straightforward (see Calculating Energy Needs, page 26). The Mifflin-St. Jeor equation has been found to be the most accurate in a variety of people. Weight is in kilograms and height is in centimeters. To convert your weight to kilograms, divide pounds by 2.2. To convert your height to centimeters, multiply your height in inches by 2.54. Then use the formula provided. The number you get is an estimate of your RMR, which is how many calories you need just to keep you alive if you were to lie in bed all day. Unless that sounds like you, the next step is to multiply the RMR by one of the activity factors listed. The final number you get will give you a good idea of the number of calories you need to maintain your weight. To lose weight at a sustainable, realistic rate, you need to subtract 500. As discussed earlier, the 500-calorie deficit should be a combination of eating less and moving more, discussed next.

- **UNDERSTAND THAT NOT ALL CALORIES ARE CREATED EQUAL** Our foods are made up of three macronutrients: carbohydrates, fats, and proteins, as well as micronutrients (including vitamins, minerals, and phyto-chemicals) and water. Carbohydrates and protein both have 4 calories per gram; fats have 9 calories per gram.

So as you can see, fat is more calorie- or energy-dense. This means it's much easier to overeat fat calories, and it's the easiest nutrient for your body to store as fat. Therefore, when selecting foods to include in your long-term weight-management plan, choose foods that your body will preferentially burn for energy or use for bodily processes before storing the excess as fat: high-fiber complex carbohydrates, and lean protein. You still need to include healthy fats in your diet for optimal health, but the emphasis should be on those foods that contain slow-burning carbohydrates and lean protein, such as whole grains, legumes, fish, lean poultry, tofu, and low-fat dairy products. These are the types of foods that will fuel your body, fill your belly, and satisfy you while keeping calories in check.

- MOVE MORE You'll want to give equal focus to your level of activity as well as the quality of your diet. As we age, we start losing valuable muscle mass, and since a pound of muscle at rest burns far more calories per hour than a pound of fat, incorporating exercise, especially strength building, is one of the best ways to combat that age-related decline in metabolism, or the number of calories you burn each day. In a later section, additional information will be provided on the components of physical activity and how to boost your current level.

- SET REALISTIC, FLEXIBLE GOALS What is reasonable and realistic in terms of goals is different for each person. However, if you set your goals too high,

you are setting yourself up for failure. You are much better off setting some long-term goals and then focusing your attention on what you can do right now by establishing daily and weekly goals. It always feels so good to check something off of a "to-do" list, so pick things that are a bit of a stretch but achievable. For example, "I will walk at a moderate pace for 30 minutes five days this week." And don't forget to be flexible. Life happens, so lose the all-or-none mentality. If your boss wants you to come into work early, or you get stuck in traffic on the way home, don't scrap your entire workout—do what you can, even if it is just 10 or 15 minutes. All-or-none and black-and-white should be removed from your healthy lifestyle mind-set. We aren't aiming for perfection, just concerted, consistent progress.

- GET 7 TO 8 HOURS OF SLEEP Studies consistently show that sleep-deprived people feel hungrier, tend to make poorer food choices, and tend to eat more (as much as 300 extra calories per day).[1] This is because lack of sleep throws your hunger hormones out of kilter, making it more likely you will overeat while also increasing levels of the stress hormone, cortisol, which causes you to store fat around your middle. Shoot for 7 to 8 hours of shut-eye per night, and try to get to bed earlier rather than sleeping in later. Consider sleep as one of the very important pieces of the weight-loss puzzle.

- MANAGE YOUR STRESS Stress can come from many areas of life and has a profound impact on weight loss and management. Just like lack of sleep, too much stress increases the levels of cortisol in your body. And while cortisol is good under some circumstances (such as preparing our bodies for flight or fight), constantly elevated levels can lead to unhealthy coping behaviors (i.e., eating when stressed), which in turn can lead to weight gain, especially around the midsection. Belly fat is particularly hard to get rid of, and is also the most harmful to health. The best way to keep cortisol in check is to maintain a healthy diet, be active every day, and take a few minutes out of each day to do something you enjoy.

- **FEED YOUR MICROBIOME** There is a lot of research focused these days on how a healthy gut influences many aspects of our health including our immune system, risk for certain diseases, and, you guessed it, our weight. The types of foods you eat can cause changes in the number and type of your gut bacteria or microbiome. Too many of the "bad bugs" and too few of the "good bugs" promotes inflammation in the body and can lead to weight gain. While this is a continuing area of research, what is known is that you can promote healthy bacteria by eating lots of fiber; fermented foods like kimchi, sauerkraut, and tempeh; and healthy fats like those found in nuts, olive oil, and fatty fish, while cutting back on saturated and trans fats, refined sugars, and processed foods. A more detailed discussion with suggestions for optimizing your gut flora can be found in A Healthy Gut and Weight Management (page 33).

DASH-ING SNACKS AROUND 150 CALORIES

1. ½ an avocado filled with ⅓ cup fat-free cottage cheese: 160 calories

2. ½ cup shelled edamame: 120 calories

3. 1 large apple with ½ tablespoon peanut butter: 150 calories

4. 1 slice whole-grain bread with 1 tablespoon hummus: 135 calories

5. 2½ cups oil-popped popcorn: 140 calories or 4½ cups air-popped popcorn: 140 calories

6. 1 mozzarella string cheese stick paired with 10 almonds: 150 calories

7. 1 hard-boiled egg and 1 small banana: 160 calories

8. ¾ cup plain low-fat (2%) Greek yogurt and ½ cup fresh strawberries: 150 calories

9. 1 ounce almonds: 160 calories

10. 1 cup baby carrots, 1 cup bell pepper strips, and 2 table-spoons hummus: 140 calories

One last piece of food for thought: Research has shown that the trifecta of sleep, stress, and gut bacteria are all interrelated when it comes to weight.[2, 3, 4]

- **TAKE STOCK OF YOUR MEDICATIONS** There are a number of medications that commonly slow down metabolism and/or contribute to weight gain. If you have recently started taking any new medications and the scale is inching upward, talk to your medical care provider and find out if there is an alternative treatment that is less likely to cause weight gain.

- **CHALLENGE YOUR HORMONES** Women seem to get the short end of the stick when it comes to weight loss. Our bodies were designed for fat storage for reproductive purposes. It is just simply harder for women to lose weight than men, and as women age and menopause creeps up, it becomes even harder. And while you can't change your biology, there are strategies that can increase your weight-loss success. One of these is to prioritize weight-bearing exercises that will build and maintain muscle mass. "The DASH Weight-Loss Meal and Exercise Plans" gives more info (see page 51). Another is to focus on the quality of your carbohydrates: Choose whole grains and where possible, swap starchy carbs like rice and pasta for beans and legumes. Additionally, I am a firm believer that knowledge is power, so simply acknowledging the weight-loss challenges that we as women face can often be a huge motivator for maintaining consistent action.

CALCULATING ENERGY NEEDS

MIFFLIN-ST. JEOR EQUATION

FOR WOMEN:
BMR = 10 × weight (kg) + 6.25 × height (cm) – 5 × age (years) – 161

FOR MEN: BMR = 10 × weight (kg) + 6.25 × height (cm) – 5 × age (years) + 5

Once you have determined your BMR, you need to multiply it by the appropriate activity factor to determine your daily calorie needs:

1.2 = sedentary
(little or no exercise)

1.375 = light activity
(light exercise/sports 1–3 days a week)

1.550 = moderate activity
(moderate exercise/sports 3–5 days a week)

1.725 = very active
(hard exercise/sports 6–7 days a week)

1.900 = extra active
(very hard exercise/sports and physical job)

Calculate Your Body Mass Index*

	BMI (KG/M^2)
Underweight	<18.5
Normal	18.5–24.9
Overweight	25.0–29.9
Obesity Class 1	30.0–34.9
Obesity Class 2	35.0–39.9
Extreme Obesity	≥40

*www.nhlbi.nih.gov/health/educational/lose_wt/BMI/bmicalc.htm

Gaining an understanding of why weight loss can be so difficult can help relieve some of the frustration and confusion and help you to be more successful. While there is no shortcut to weight loss, you can make the process easier with a few simple changes to your behavior.

Behavior Modification Tips and Tricks

Successful weight loss and weight management involves more than the types and amounts of the foods you eat. It also involves the thousands of decisions we make each day that influence those choices. Many of these are automatic habits ingrained in our subconscious that may or may not be to our benefit. For example, maybe when you come home from work you walk through the kitchen and automatically grab a soda. Behavior modification for weight loss involves self-awareness of target behaviors and outcomes, and creating new patterns of action as needed to create healthy patterns of long-term lifestyle change. The following section includes a few options to consider as you build your own healthy and sustainable lifestyle:

- FIND YOUR INNER MOTIVATION As mentioned earlier, it is hard to make lasting change without a meaningful reason or two. Don't embark on weight loss without getting really clear on why you want to do it. Consider writing your top three reasons down and putting them where you see them every day such as on the bathroom mirror or in your day planner.

- WRITE DOWN YOUR GOALS Along with your inner motivation, you will want to set two or three S.M.A.R.T. goals: Specific, Measurable, Achievable, Realistic/relevant, and Time-bound. For example, lose 5 percent of your body weight in six months, or walk a 5K race in

June. Write these down along with your motivations for change. See page 31 for an example of a S.M.A.R.T. goal.

- **KNOW YOUR TRIGGERS** It's incredibly insightful to become aware of your food and exercise triggers, good and bad. Does the sight of French fries on a TV commercial send you headed out the door to the drive-through? Does rain make you want to ditch your workout? Does a bad day at work infuse your evening workout with intensity? Start noticing and naming, then list two or three strategies to overcome each negative trigger and promote positive action that keeps you moving forward. For example, if it is raining, do "house walking" instead. If food commercials make you crave unhealthy foods, get up and move while they are on or leave the room. If you had a bad day at work, use the stress as a motivator for a high-intensity workout instead of a reason to indulge in high-sugar, high-fat, or high-calorie foods. I have a punching bag hanging in my garage for those stressful days and I feel so much better using physical activity as my outlet.

- **RECOGNIZE HUNGER VERSUS APPETITE** Hunger is a physiological need, while appetite is a psychological yearning. Notice if you are truly hungry or if it is simply appetite. If you truly are physically hungry, have a healthy snack or start prepping and cooking your meal.

- **FOCUS ON PROGRESS NOT PERFECTION** Sustained consistent action is the key to long-term lifestyle change.

There are going to be setbacks—in fact there will be many of them along the way. Decide you are "in it" for the long haul and don't let slip ups derail your whole plan. Simply "clean the slate" and move forward.

- **PRACTICE MINDFULNESS** When you eat, focus on the distinct flavors and textures of your foods. How do different foods affect your hunger and fullness? Being mindful can help you tune in to your body's hunger and fullness cues. This is a skill that takes practice, so be patient with yourself as you become a more intuitive eater.

- **DOWNSIZE YOUR PLATES AND BOWLS** A simple portion-control behavior modification technique is to use smaller plates (about 8 to 10 inches in diameter) and smaller bowls. Your glass size makes a difference, too: People tend to serve more when short, wide glasses are used than tall, narrow ones.

- **KEEP A FOOD DIARY** Food journaling is a proven weight-loss and weight-management technique. If you have to log or write down everything you eat and drink, it can help you identify patterns and make you aware of how much you are eating. Consider keeping a food journal for a week or two, until you have established a good pattern. If you find it motivates you and keeps you on track, consider keeping up this habit.

- **EAT SLOWLY WITHOUT DISTRACTIONS** Did you know it takes at least 20 minutes for the signals in your stomach to reach your brain and tell it you have had enough to eat? Many of us are guilty of eating too quickly, which means we often eat more than we need. Do this: Set a kitchen timer or the timer on your phone for 20 minutes and practice stretching out each of your meals for at least this length of time. Notice how you feel in terms of hunger and fullness.

- **CONTROL YOUR ENVIRONMENT** Do you eat while standing in the kitchen, driving in your car, or while watching TV? Consider eating only while sitting down at the kitchen or dining room table.

- **MAKE HEALTHY FOODS VISIBLE AND PUT LESS HEALTHY FOODS AWAY** Keep a bowl of fruit and other healthy snacks on the kitchen counter. A recent study found that people who kept a bowl of fruit on the counter instead of cereal or candy had a lower BMI.[5] This also applies to the fridge and pantry: Put chopped veggies, lean proteins, and low-fat dairy front and center at eye level in the fridge, and whole grains, nuts, and legumes at the front of the pantry.

- **DRINK WATER** Dehydration is often confused with hunger. Ensure you are drinking enough water each day. There is no hard-and-fast rule for this; however, 64 ounces per day is a good amount to aim for. If you don't enjoy the taste of water, pick up an inexpensive fruit infuser water bottle or simply add pieces of citrus or berries to your water.

- **FOLLOW THE 80/20 RULE** No foods are 100 percent off limits, but spend your calories wisely. Many people find that

---

10 WAYS TO BURN 100 CALORIES

(Values are approximate based on a 150-pound person.)

1. Bowl: 30 minutes

2. Cook a meal: 45 minutes

3. Walk the dog: 26 minutes

4. Wash and clean your car: 20 minutes

5. Mow the lawn: 20 minutes

6. Practice yoga: 20 minutes

7. Go for a bike ride: 23 minutes

8. Mop the floors: 20 minutes

9. Golf, carrying clubs: 15 minutes

10. Swim at moderate intensity: 15 minutes

---

choosing healthy foods 80 percent of the time and less healthy foods 20 percent of the time gives them the proper balance of nourishing foods interspersed with reasonable treats.

- **EAT BREAKFAST** You have heard this one many times before, but starting out your day with a healthy, balanced breakfast refuels you after an overnight fast, keeps your blood sugar steady and energy up, and helps your concentration. A nutritious breakfast can also keep you from overeating at lunchtime. Ditch the typical refined carb–heavy American

7 WEIGHT-LOSS MYTHS AND FACTS

1. **MYTH:** Losing weight is a linear process.
   FACT: Your weight will fluctuate up and down a few pounds. This is normal and as long as the general trend is downward you will succeed over the long term.

2. **MYTH:** Carbohydrates in grains and fruit make you fat.
   FACT: Complex carbohydrates in grains are an excellent source of slow-burning energy, fiber, vitamins, and minerals. Refined carbohydrates are linked to weight gain but whole grains are not. Fruits contain sugar, but they also contain fiber, vitamins, and minerals and should be included in your diet.

3. **MYTH:** Fast food is off limits.
   FACT: You don't have to give up eating out, but you do need to make nutritious choices. Most fast-food restaurants offer grilled meats and salads—just make sure that dressings and toppings are on the side, and check the nutrition information for calories, fat, and sodium.

4. **MYTH:** Going gluten-free is the solution to weight loss.
   FACT: Many gluten-free products are highly processed and contain far less fiber and more calories and carbohydrates than their gluten-containing counterparts. Gluten-free foods are not healthier and if you don't have celiac or gluten sensitivity, you don't need them.

5. **MYTH:** Detoxing and juicing are good ways to lose weight.
   FACT: There is no clear and consistent evidence that juicing or detoxing will help with sustained weight loss. Juicing removes most of the fiber from fruits and vegetables so you are left with a nonfilling, caloric drink.

6. **MYTH:** Cutting fat from your diet helps you lose weight.
   FACT: A no-fat diet doesn't taste good, so people tend to overcompensate and eat more. Eating healthy fats (avocado, nuts, salmon, etc.) boosts satisfaction, lowers inflammation, and keeps metabolism up.

7. **MYTH:** The more calories you cut, the faster you lose weight.
   FACT: If you cut out too many calories, your metabolism will slow to conserve fat—a protective mechanism in times of famine. Women should not eat fewer than 1,200 calories per day, and men should not go below 1,500 calories per day.

SELF-COMPASSION AND WEIGHT LOSS

Losing weight is hard, often triggers negative emotions, and for most dieters, involves judging oneself as good or bad, or comparing oneself with others. Negative self-talk is not only demoralizing, but it can also set you up for overeating. Self-compassion on the other hand involves relating to yourself kindly, like you would with a friend or small child, with care and concern. Self-compassion is strongly associated with less anxiety and depression, and more optimism and motivation, which can boost your weight-loss success. Self-compassion researcher Dr. Kristin Neff provides the following tips for changing the way you relate to yourself:[6]

- Progress, not perfection: When you find you are being hard on yourself, remind yourself that weight loss is a process and change doesn't happen overnight.
- Watch your words: Avoid negative statements like "I cheated" or "I am a failure"—any negative terms you wouldn't use with a small child or friend. Notice when you think them and replace them with more supportive terms like "maybe that wasn't the best choice," "this is hard," "next time I will take more time to choose something that fits with my goals."
- Examine what happened: Keeping a daily journal in which you process the difficult events of your day through a lens of self-compassion can help make kindness and mindfulness part of your daily life.

Habit change comes so much easier when you are more relaxed and accepting. Take some time for your self-compassion practice today.

A S.M.A.R.T. Goal Example

GOAL	Improve my level of fitness
HOW I WILL ACHIEVE THIS	Walk 3 days a week at a moderate pace for 30 minutes.
WHEN I WILL ACHIEVE THIS	I will start today and continue this routine as part of my healthy long-term lifestyle.
CONTINGENCY PLAN	If it is raining, I will "house-walk" for 30 minutes or go to the mall and walk. If I have to work late, I will choose another day to complete my 30 minutes.

breakfast and opt for a meal that includes ample protein, one to two servings of fruits or veggies, and a serving of fiber-rich grains.

- **PREPARE YOUR OWN MEALS** Preparing the majority of your own meals does a number of positive things: Cooking burns calories, preparing your own foods lets you control the types and amounts of ingredients, and preparing your own meals saves you money.

- **MOVE EVERY 30 MINUTES** In addition to purposeful exercise, simply moving more during the day is an easy behavioral strategy to implement. Research shows that even if we do 30 or 60 minutes of physical activity each day but sit for the rest of the day, health risks for certain chronic diseases are still elevated. If you spend most of the day at your computer, get up and move at least every 30 minutes. Download a browser extension or app that you can set to remind you to take breaks.

- **INCORPORATE INCENTIVES** Consider having a list of nonfood incentives to support your behavior change. Rewards or incentives can be anything and don't have to cost any money. For example, an afternoon reading a book, a hot bath, a new workout top, or that new kitchen tool you have been eyeing.

Adopting a healthier lifestyle involves more than just making changes to the types and amounts of foods that you eat. Lifestyle change over time takes consistent and sustained action, and whether we achieve our goals depends on how we make them, on our mind-set, and on the strategies we put in place to maintain our motivation and encourage our success.

Physical Activity

Being physically active is an essential part of a healthy lifestyle and it comes with so many immediate and long-term benefits to your overall well-being. Activity and exercise reduce your risk for a number of chronic diseases including high blood pressure, high cholesterol, heart disease, stroke, type 2 diabetes, osteoporosis, and certain

Healthy Food Swaps

INSTEAD OF THIS . . .	CHOOSE THIS . . .
Butter on bread	Smashed avocado on bread
Sour cream	Low-fat (2%) Greek yogurt
Processed salad dressing	Extra-virgin olive oil and vinegar
Cream-based dips	Salsa
Soda	Sparkling water
Chips	Air-popped popcorn
Sugary breakfast cereal	Steel-cut oats
White rice	Brown rice
White pasta	Spiralized vegetable noodles
Iceberg lettuce	Spinach, arugula, or kale

A HEALTHY GUT AND WEIGHT MANAGEMENT

Four ways to feed your good bacteria

1. **PREBIOTICS** Prebiotics are plant fiber compounds that pass through your GI tract undigested and encourage the growth of good bacteria by feeding them. Good sources include asparagus, Jerusalem artichoke, jicama, garlic, bananas, and onions.

2. **PROBIOTICS** Probiotics are a type of good bacteria similar to the types found in your GI tract. Good sources include fermented foods like kimchi, tempeh, yogurt, sauerkraut, kefir, and miso. You can also use dietary supplements.

3. **FIBER** Fiber found in fruits, vegetables, and whole grains helps promote the growth of friendly bacteria. The DASH diet is rich in fiber and can help you to meet the recommended 25 to 35 grams per day.

4. **HEALTHY FATS** Consume more omega-3 fatty acids such as those found in fatty fish and flaxseeds, and monounsaturated fats such as those found in avocado and extra-virgin olive oil.

---

cancers. Physical activity also contributes to healthy aging by improving brain function and protecting memory and thinking skills, and by reducing the risk of falls by offsetting the decline in muscle mass with age. Mentally, being active can raise your self-esteem, boost your mood, and ward off depression. Importantly, activity, especially strength exercises and higher intensity aerobic activity, can protect against the decline in metabolic rate that comes with weight loss. In other words, as you lose weight, you won't have to keep continually cutting calories to maintain your loss if you engage in regular exercise.

The two main types of exercise are aerobic and strength building, or anaerobic. Aerobic or cardiovascular exercises benefit your heart and lungs and include walking, swimming, biking, mowing the lawn, running, jogging, and other exercises involving your large muscle groups. Strength exercises build and maintain muscle and include activities such as using resistance bands, doing body-weight exercise, and/or lifting weights.

The US Department of Health and Human Services *2018 Physical Activity Guidelines for Americans* provides the following guidelines for adults:

- **AVOID INACTIVITY** Some activity is better than none, and all activity has health benefits.

- **AEROBIC ACTIVITY** For substantial health benefits and weight management, adults

BEFRIEND FIBER

A high-fiber diet, like DASH, can help you to manage your weight through its ability to keep you full longer, which prevents overeating and hunger between meals. Because DASH is higher in dietary fiber than the standard American diet, take care to add the recommended amounts of vegetables, fruits, and whole grains slowly (such as over the course of a week) to allow your body to adjust. Remember to drink plenty of water to avoid constipation.

WHAT IS FIBER?

Fiber is the structural part of plant foods such as fruits, vegetables, and grains that our bodies cannot digest. There are two main categories of fiber: soluble and insoluble.

- **Soluble fiber:** Dissolves to form a gummy gel. It can slow down the passage of food from the stomach, keeping blood-sugar levels steady. Soluble fiber can also lower cholesterol and the risk for heart disease. Sources include legumes (beans, lentils, and peas), oats and oat bran, barley, fruits (bananas, apples, pears, etc.), and vegetables.

- **Insoluble fiber:** Is often referred to as roughage because it doesn't dissolve in water. Its ability to hold on to water can produce softer, bulkier stools to regulate bowel movements. Evidence suggests insoluble fiber may reduce the risk for intestinal cancer. Sources include whole-grain products, rolled oats, brown rice, buckwheat, bran, nuts, corn, fruits with edible peels or seeds (carrots, berries, apples, pears etc.), vegetables, and cereals.

HOW MUCH DO I NEED?

- Men under the age of 50 need 38 grams per day, and men ages 51 to 70 years need 30 grams; women under the age of 50 need 25 grams per day, and women ages 51 to 70 years need 21 grams. Ten to 15 grams should come from soluble fiber.

- In order for a food to be labeled as "high fiber" it must contain 5 grams or more of dietary fiber per serving.

should do at least 150 minutes (2 hours 30 minutes) a week of moderate-intensity activity, or 75 minutes (1 hour 15 minutes) a week of vigorous-intensity activity, or a combination of moderate and vigorous-intensity aerobic activity.

For even greater health benefits and as part of a weight-loss program, adults should do one of the following: Increase moderate-intensity activity to 300 minutes (5 hours) each week, or increase vigorous-intensity activity to 150 minutes (2 hours 30 minutes) each week. For weight control, the guidelines suggest that vigorous-intensity activity is far more time efficient than moderate-intensity activity.

- STRENGTHEN MUSCLES Do muscle-strengthening activities (such as resistance bands or lifting weights) that are moderate or high intensity and involve all major muscle groups on 2 or more days of the week.

- FLEXIBILITY AND STRETCHING Flexibility activities and stretching are also important parts of a fitness plan. Flexibility determines your range of motion, or how far you can bend and stretch muscles and ligaments. Being flexible can enhance postural stability and balance and stretching can improve flexibility. Include both a warm-up and a cool-down that includes stretching and movement that extends muscles through their range of motion to improve flexibility and reduce the risk of injury.

One of the easiest and safest ways to get started with activity is to begin walking at a moderate-intensity pace, fast enough to get your heart pumping while still allowing you to talk comfortably. And although brisk walking is safe for most people, there are certain cases in which you should receive medical clearance before exercising. Health experts suggest you talk with your doctor before you start exercising if you have heart disease, cancer, type 1 or 2 diabetes, kidney disease, or arthritis. In addition, the American College of Sports Medicine recommends that you see a doctor to receive medical clearance if two or more of the following apply:[7]

- You are older than 35 years
- You have a family history of heart disease before age 60
- You smoke or quit smoking in the past 6 months
- You don't normally exercise for at least 30 minutes most days of the week
- You are significantly overweight
- You have high blood pressure or cholesterol
- You have type 1 or 2 diabetes, or impaired blood glucose tolerance

You might be thinking: "How can I fit exercise into an already overloaded schedule?" It isn't easy, but with creativity and determination, it can be done. An active lifestyle should be one of everyone's top priorities in life as being healthy allows us to be our best—for ourselves, and for our family and friends. Some tips for making time for activity include:

- **SCHEDULE EXERCISE SESSIONS** Mark breaks throughout the day in your day planner or calendar just as you would other commitments. Accumulate 10 minutes at a time as you can and combine activity with other tasks. For example, while talking on the phone, stand up and do leg raises or squats. When walking the dog, do it briskly and include a few hills if you can.

- **HAVE YOUR WORKOUT CLOTHES AND SHOES LAID OUT THE NIGHT BEFORE** And without cutting into your sleep, set your alarm 30 minutes earlier and go for a brisk walk.

- **MIX SOCIALIZING WITH EXERCISING** Grab a friend and go for a bike ride instead of going to the movies; walk with coworkers at lunchtime; take a dance class.

- **CHOOSE AN ACTIVITY YOU ENJOY** If you hate running, don't do it! Experiment until you find the exercise that works best for you.

Finding Fiber in Foods

FOOD	SERVING	TOTAL FIBER (GRAMS)	SOLUBLE (GRAMS)	INSOLUBLE (GRAMS)
Brussels sprouts	½ cup	2.8	1.7	1.1
Carrots	1 medium	2.3	1.1	1.2
Apple	1 small	2.8	1.0	1.8
Black beans	½ cup	6.1	2.4	3.7
Wheat germ	3 tbsp	3.9	0.7	3.2
Flaxseed	1 tbsp	3.3	1.1	2.2
Oatmeal	⅓ cup dry	2.7	1.4	1.3
Wheat bran	½ cup	12.3	1.0	11.3
Kale	½ cup	2.5	0.7	1.8
Sweet potato	½ cup	4.0	1.8	2.2

- **CUT DOWN ON MEDIA** As discussed earlier, keep a 24-hour time diary and replace time spent surfing the web with exercise.

- **WORK OUT EFFICIENTLY** Choose a form of exercise you can do almost anywhere and focus on higher intensity activity to get the most bang for your buck: Interval training, body-weight exercises, and speed walking are all great choices.

- **LOSE THE ALL-OR-NONE MENTALITY** Some exercise is better than none and all activity counts. Always be thinking of ways you can fit in snippets of activity throughout your day.

Finally, remember to simply get up and move for a couple of minutes after every 30 to 60 minutes of sitting. Even if you include 30 minutes or more of purposeful exercise each day, sitting for prolonged periods of time increases your health risks for chronic diseases. Pages 62–67 will include a simple physical activity plan to accompany the meal plans with tips for modifying the types and amounts of activity for varying degrees of fitness.

Building a Support System

The journey of weight loss can be a difficult and lonely one, and it can be even harder if your family isn't on board. Explain to your family and friends you are embarking on the DASH diet for weight loss and let them know why it is important to you. Discuss how following DASH is an ideal choice for the whole family and is an eating plan full of great tasting foods. Let them know the recipes in this book are family favorites given a DASH boost of nutrition so that everyone's health will benefit. Aim to involve the whole family in meal planning and talk about ways to give favorite family recipes a makeover. If you are met with objections over desired snack foods and treats by your children and/or spouse, a good strategy is to ask each member for a list of several "treat" items they want to keep in the house. Then designate special areas of the pantry and fridge for these items that are slightly out of your view, while putting healthy choices like cut-up vegetables and fruits, and low-fat dairy products front and center. This will help avoid temptation on your part, while also encouraging your family to reach for the more nutritious snack options.

Enlisting the family in physical activity is also a great way to spend more time together while improving everyone's fitness. After dinner, instead of watching TV, take a walk together. On the weekends organize a family bike ride, go swimming in the summer, plant a family garden, or go hiking together.

And while loving friends and family are the best support, there are cases where you will be met with jealousy, anger, food "pushers," and those wishing to sabotage your plan. The best course of action in this case is to research support groups in your area or online, and find a group of like-minded people who will encourage you in your lifestyle changes.

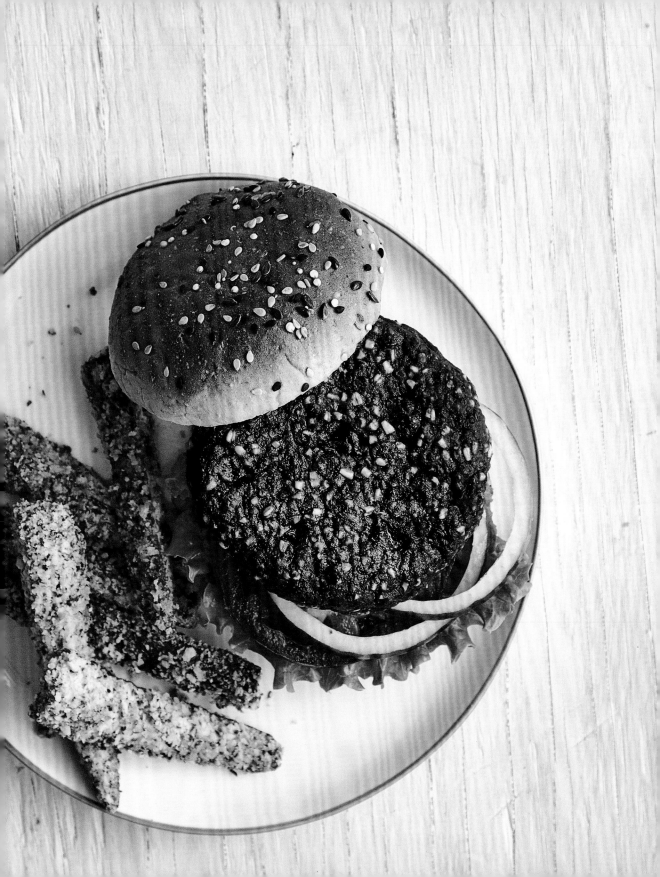

Setting Yourself Up for Success

Now that you have learned the basics of the DASH eating plan for weight loss, the foundational concepts of weight management, the components of a balanced physical activity plan, and ways to incorporate positive behavior change strategies, you are ready for what I think is the best part: setting up your kitchen and learning how to maximize your efficiency so you can fuel yourself with nutritious foods even when your life and schedule are busy. With a quick pantry reorganization, simple food swaps, and suggestions for time-saving kitchen tools, you can transform your kitchen so that it is more inspiring, and your cooking will become easier and healthier automatically.

Kitchen Cleanout

Because healthy eating following the DASH plan is a certain type of lifestyle, you have to physically set up your environment to help you more easily accomplish your wellness goals. Just like with any lifestyle choice, your mind and body benefit from external cues to help guide you. A bowl of fruit on the counter, a fridge with cut-up vegetables, and a well-ordered pantry stocked with nutritious staples are all cues that can make a big difference in your actions.

There are four areas to focus on when setting up a healthy kitchen: the pantry, the freezer/refrigerator, your spice cabinet, and the counter. A kitchen review and cleanout can seem overwhelming, bring up emotions, and feel like a lot of work. However, the process can be made less painful, quicker, and more efficient by using the following tips:

1. **PLAN MEALS FOR THE NEXT 2 TO 3 DAYS BEFORE YOU START THE PANTRY/FREEZER/REFRIGERATOR CLEANOUT** Making changes in your kitchen can be unsettling, especially if you don't want to waste food or can't donate it because the package is opened or the food is partially used. Planning out a few days' worth of meals can also ease some of the stress associated with purging your pantry, and we all feel better when we have a plan. Set these foods aside now.

2. **ORGANIZE YOUR PANTRY** Start by removing all of the foods from your pantry and cupboards. Designate counter space to go through each item. It's crucial to involve your partner and children in this step to avoid anger and resentment. Have each family member choose a few favorites that they want to keep in the house. Designate a shelf or cupboard for storing these items, such as a "snack" zone for the kids, or a "treat" zone for your partner.

   Next, to determine which items stay or go, read expiration dates and food labels. If any items are expired, discard them. After this, do a global review and move all of the "obvious" less healthy choices to the side. By "obvious" I mean things like bags of cookies, chips, boxed meals like macaroni and cheese, sugar-filled breakfast cereals, and so on. To determine which foods stay and which go, read the food label and ingredient list and remove items high in sodium and/or sugar, with more than ten ingredients, and those with manmade hydrogenated fats. Keep in mind that removing unhealthy foods from your environment makes it so much easier to eat well. When you are finished, clean the shelves and organize your pantry with healthy ingredients front and center. If your shelves are a bit bare at this point, not to worry as after the cleanout you will be restocking with healthy essentials.

3. **ORGANIZE YOUR REFRIGERATOR AND FREEZER** Repeat the same process with the items in your refrigerator and freezer. Foods you will want to donate or use up include processed meats, high-sodium bottled sauces, sugar-sweetened beverages, packaged frozen dinners, frozen vegetables with sauces or added

ingredients, frozen fruits with added sugars, and meats and fish with breading or added sauces. Check the labels of your condiments and consider using up or getting rid of those that are high in sugar and/or sodium.

4. **ORGANIZE YOUR SPICE CABINET**
Spices and herbs have negligible calories, are full of nutrients, and add flavor to your foods naturally without the use of salt or added fats. Remove all of your spices and seasoning from your cabinet so you can take stock of what you have. As a general rule, whole spices will stay fresh for about four years (cloves, peppercorns, cinnamon sticks), ground spices for two to three years (nutmeg, cinnamon, turmeric), dried herbs one to three years (basil, oregano, parsley), and extracts about four years. Despite these long shelf lives, you will get more flavor by changing your dried spices and herbs every 12 months or so. Make a list of what you have and smell them to see if they are still pungent. In the next section on stocking your kitchen, I've included a list of essential spices every cook should have in their pantry.

5. **ORGANIZE YOUR COUNTERTOPS**
Cluttered countertops and disorder in the kitchen may make you more apt to choose less healthy foods, according to a number of research studies. One recent study published in *Environment and Behavior* set up two kitchens: One was neat and tidy while the other was strewn with mail, newspapers, and dirty dishes.[1] Over a hundred women were recruited to participate in the study and were told to wait alone in either the messy or clean kitchen for another person to arrive, and to help themselves to snacks (cookies, carrots, and crackers). The researchers also asked some of the women to write about a time when they felt out of control, while others wrote about a time they were in control. The results? The women in the messy kitchens who entered with negative thoughts in mind ate 100 more calories from cookies than the women in the tidy kitchen. What this study shows us is that if you come home from a crazy stressful day of work, and your kitchen is a mess, you are more likely to choose unhealthy foods and overeat them.

A few steps you can take to declutter your kitchen include keeping your countertops clear and avoiding the temptation to use them to place your keys, the mail, magazines, dirty dishes, and any other miscellaneous items. Store any nonessential appliances in your cabinets so that your countertops are functional for your cooking. Allow yourself to have one messy "junk" drawer to stash those miscellaneous items. It's also important to assess your workflow: Does it make the most sense for your cutting boards and knives to be next to the kitchen sink? What appliances do you use daily and are they conveniently located? Are your spices within easy reach? Finally, have a morning and evening kitchen ritual: For example, before you leave for work, empty and rinse the coffeepot; at the end of the day, wipe down the counters and empty the dishwasher.

Now that you have taken stock of the foods you have on hand and organized your kitchen, it's time to restock with healthy cooking staples.

Stocking Your Kitchen with DASH-Friendly Foods

The next step in setting up your healthy kitchen is to restock it with staples and minimally processed foods. This does not have to be done all at once and you can begin by choosing one or two categories to swap out each week. For example, one week refresh your dried spices and herbs, and the next swap out white flour for whole-wheat flour and white rice for brown rice. This will make the transition less overwhelming and easier on your budget. Here are some recommendations for the types of foods and staples to keep on hand, but you shouldn't take this as a prescription. Instead, customize this list based on your personal food preferences:

PANTRY

- **GRAINS** Choose fiber-filled whole grains like quinoa, barley, brown rice, wild rice, whole-wheat pasta, rolled oats, steel-cut oats, buckwheat, and millet.
- **BEANS** This nutritional powerhouse is budget friendly, and a smart food for weight loss. Stock a variety of canned and dried beans and other legumes, such as lentils, black beans, chickpeas, cannellini beans, kidney beans, and pinto beans.
- **NUTS AND SEEDS** No-salt, no-added-oil nuts like almonds, walnuts, pistachios, and pecans, as well as seeds such as pumpkin, sunflower, flax, and chia are perfect for incorporating into baked goods, sprinkling on foods, snacking, and using in recipes.
- **OILS AND VINEGAR** Choose healthy fats like extra-virgin olive oil and avocado oil, and keep balsamic and red wine vinegar on hand.
- **NUT BUTTERS** Go for natural varieties without added sugars or salt. Peanut, walnut, cashew, almond, and tahini are all great choices.
- **SNACKS** Air-popped popcorn, no-sugar-added dried fruit and freeze-dried fruit, dried vegetable chips like kale and beet, and whole-grain crackers all make nutritious snack choices.
- **FLOURS** Choose whole-wheat, whole-wheat pastry, oat, chickpea, almond, and quinoa flours for baking.
- **SWEETENERS** Use unrefined sweeteners in moderation including honey, maple syrup, and molasses and consider stocking stevia, a no-calorie plant-derived sweetener.
- **VEGETABLES** Potatoes, sweet potatoes, onions, garlic
- **FRESH FRUITS** Bananas

REFRIGERATOR

- **MILK** Low-fat or fat-free milk or plant-based milk
- **YOGURT AND CHEESES** Low-fat (2%) or nonfat (0%) Greek yogurt, cottage cheese, ricotta cheese, and shredded cheeses
- **EGGS**
- **FRESH VEGETABLES** Baby lettuces, tomatoes, mushrooms, broccoli, zucchini, carrots, cabbage, celery
- **FRESH FRUITS** Avocadoes, apples, citrus fruits, berries

FREEZER

- **VEGETABLES** Spinach, kale, green beans, green peas, riced cauliflower, butternut squash
- **FRUITS** No-sugar-added strawberries, peaches, cherries, blueberries, raspberries
- **PROTEINS** Chicken breasts, fish, lean pork, lean beef

READING A FOOD LABEL

Reading food labels when you are shopping will help you to make informed food choices and become a savvy shopper. You may have noticed a change in food labels recently, as the US Food and Drug Administration has updated labeling to be much easier to read. Some of the key changes include larger type and an emphasis on key nutrients. The new labels let you easily find out which foods are good sources of dietary fiber, vitamin D, calcium, iron, and potassium, and those that are lower in saturated fat, sodium, and added sugars and have 0 grams trans fat.

To read a food label follow these quick tips:

- Check the servings per container and serving size, and remember to check your portion size compared with the serving size listed. If the label serving is 1 cup and you eat 2 cups, remember to double the calories and other nutrients listed.
- Check the total calories to find out how many are in a single serving.
- Limit saturated fat, trans fat, sodium, and added sugars, as eating less of these can reduce your risk for chronic diseases. Limit saturated fats to less than 10% of total calories, keep trans fats at 0 grams, limit sodium to 2,300 mg per day, and limit added sugars to less than 10% of total calories.
- Eat more dietary fiber, vitamin D, calcium, and potassium, all of which are needed to maintain health including a healthy blood pressure.
- Check the ingredient list. Ingredients are listed in descending order by weight. If a product lists high-fructose corn syrup as the first ingredient, then it is the ingredient in the largest amount.

DRIED HERBS AND SPICES

- **HERBS** Basil, rosemary, thyme, oregano, dill, parsley, sage
- **SWEET SPICES** Cinnamon, nutmeg, ginger, cardamom, cloves
- **SAVORY SPICES** Black pepper, garlic powder, onion powder, mustard, cayenne, cumin, turmeric, curry, paprika, chili powder
- Vanilla extract
- Salt

Cooking Tools

Ensuring your kitchen is equipped with essential tools will make cooking so much easier, faster, and efficient. If you are just starting out, begin with these kitchen basics, adding essentials as your budget allows.

ESSENTIALS

- **CAN OPENER** Electric or manual
- **INSTANT-READ THERMOMETER** For food safety, the internal temperature of meats should always be checked to ensure they are properly cooked.
- **TIMER** Most cell phones have timers, too.
- **OVEN MITT AND HOT PADS** Cloth or silicone to protect your hands from being burned
- **KITCHEN TOWELS AND DISHCLOTHS** For cleaning up, drying dishes, and wiping down spills

- **FOIL** For easy cleanup and for packet cooking.
- **STORAGE CONTAINERS** High-quality storage containers are essential for storing leftovers and for packing lunch. Glass containers are microwave-, dishwasher-, freezer-safe, and BPA-free. Aim for an assortment of sizes: 1-cup, 2-cup, 4-cup.
- **PARCHMENT PAPER** For lining sheet pans and packet cooking
- **RESEALABLE PLASTIC BAGS** Sandwich- and freezer-size bags for storing leftover ingredients in the refrigerator or freezer.

PREPARATION AND COOKING TOOLS

- **DRY AND LIQUID MEASURING CUPS** You will want measuring cups for both dry and wet ingredients. Nesting stainless steel cups work well for dry ingredients while a large (4-cup) microwave-safe glass cup works well for liquids.
- **MEASURING SPOONS** Oval types are more likely to fit into spice jars.
- **ASSORTED KNIVES** A good-quality chef's knife with an 8- to 10-inch blade and a small paring knife should cover your chopping needs.
- **WHISK** A wire whisk is great for combining dry baking ingredients, beating eggs, and mixing sauces and vinaigrettes.
- **GRATER** A box grater is the most versatile, with options to shred, shave, and zest.

- **VEGETABLE PEELER** Y-peelers are easier to handle than the swivel peeler alternative, and faster to use.
- **COLANDER** Choose one with feet on the bottom so that when you drain your pasta or other foods they don't sit in the puddle of water.
- **CUTTING BOARD(S)** Wooden boards tend to be more sanitary and are less likely to dull your knives. If you can afford it, buy two: one for meats and one for vegetables and fruits.
- **SPATULA** A multifunction tool, spatulas are used for stirring sauces, scrambling eggs, turning, and spreading. Silicone types are heat-resistant.
- **STIRRING SPOON AND SLOTTED SPOON** Choose ones that are durable, heat-resistant, dishwasher-safe, and won't scratch pots and pans.
- **MIXING BOWLS** Choose nested ones in an assortment of sizes. These will be used for baking, marinating, sauces, and seasonings.
- **POTATO MASHER** One with a curved head will allow you to get into the corners of bowls and pots.

COOKWARE AND BAKEWARE

- **SKILLET WITH LID** One of the most versatile stovetop tools for cooking nearly everything, a skillet is used for frying, searing, sautéing, and browning. Nonstick varieties need less oil to coat the pan; cast-iron can go from stovetop to oven.
- **SAUTÉ PAN WITH LID** With higher sides than a skillet and a wide flat bottom, a sauté pan is perfect for cooking greens, sauces, and braising meats.
- **SAUCEPAN WITH LID** Small saucepans are perfect for smaller portions of soups and sauces while medium sizes are suited for larger batches.
- **6- TO 8-QUART STOCKPOT WITH LID** For large portions of soups, stews, ears of corn, pasta, and sauces.
- **21 × 15-INCH OR LARGER RIMMED BAKING SHEET** For roasting and baking food in the oven including vegetables, cookies, homemade fries, and meats.
- **MUFFIN TIN** Essential for baking sweet and savory muffins; choose a nonstick type.
- **CASSEROLE DISH** A large deep dish with high edges for baking and serving one-dish meals.
- **BROILER PAN** Much thicker than a baking sheet and meant to be used under the high heat of the broiler, this type of pan is used when you want your food to have a crusty, browned top.

APPLIANCES

- **HIGH-SPEED BLENDER** For making smoothies, dips, sauces, and pureeing soups. Choose one with at least 1,000 watts of power so you can easily process a variety of ingredients.

Fun Nonessential Cooking Tools

In addition to essential tools and equipment, there are countless nice-to-have items that can make cooking faster and easier. Here are a few tools you might consider:

- **SLOW COOKER** A slow cooker is great for the busy cook who wants to have dinner waiting after a long day of work. Slow cookers are also perfect for big batches of oats and grains.

- **RICE COOKER** A wonderful, time-saving appliance for cooking grains, including rice, quinoa, and oats.

- **MULTIFUNCTION COOKER** A multifunction cooker can take the place of several appliances and save counter space while being very functional. A typical multifunction cooker takes the place of a rice cooker, pressure cooker, slow cooker, and yogurt maker.

- **IMMERSION BLENDER** A handheld immersion blender makes pureeing soups and sauces a breeze and avoids the additional steps of transferring foods to a blender to puree in batches.

- **SPIRALIZER** A useful tool for quickly making vegetable noodles out of zucchini, beets, and other vegetables.

- **FOOD PROCESSOR** If you have a high-powered blender, then you probably don't need a food processor. This appliance might be nice if you want to make your own nut butters, chop large amounts of anything, and want to make homemade dips like hummus. Depending on the model, you can use it to shred, chop, and puree.

- **RAMEKINS** Ramekins are small glazed ceramic dishes used for baking and serving various dishes. Perfectly portioned, 3-ounce, 4.5-ounce, 7-ounce, and 10-ounce types are nice for making single servings of sides, muffins, desserts, and casseroles.

- **TOFU PRESS** For removing the water from tofu instead of using stacked plates.

- **GARLIC PRESS** A nice, time-saving tool.

- **KITCHEN SHEARS** For cutting up a whole chicken and other meats, stripping herbs, cutting dried fruits, and cutting vegetables.

- **MICROPLANE GRATER** For small tasks that require a fine grater such as zesting and grating garlic.

- **SALAD SPINNER** Great for quick and easy cleaning of greens.

- **OIL MISTER** A small refillable canister that you fill with the oil of your choice, an oil mister can be used as an economical alternative to aerosol spray cans for greasing pans or misting salad greens.

Healthiest Cooking Techniques

A dash of salt here, a splash of oil there, and before you know it your healthy ingredients have been transformed into a high-salt, high-fat, calorie-heavy meal. Eating well involves more than selecting and preparing fresh, nutritious ingredients; it also involves using cooking techniques that retain the most nutrients while requiring the minimal use of added fats, oils, and salt. The following list describes some of the healthiest cooking techniques you can use to cook flavorful foods without unnecessary extras:

Sautéing

What it is and why it is healthy: This technique quickly cooks by searing, and while it requires some oil in the pan, it should be only a small amount. If you have a good-quality nonstick pan, you won't need to add any fat and can use cooking spray, low-sodium broth, or water in place of the oil.

What it is good for: Grains like rice and quinoa, thin-cut vegetables like bell pepper strips, julienned carrots, and snow peas, and bite-size pieces of meats.

Stir-frying

What it is and why it is healthy: This method involves quickly cooking foods over high heat while constantly stirring. Stir-frying requires the use of only a small amount of oil, and because vegetables are cooked quickly, this is a good technique for maintaining nutrients.

What it is good for: Lean, tender cuts of meats, vegetables, and tofu.

Roasting and Baking

What it is and why it is healthy: Both techniques involve cooking foods using the oven's dry heat without the use of added fats or oils. Foods can be roasted on a baking sheet or in a roasting pan or baked covered or uncovered.

What it is good for: Muffins, breads, desserts, seafood, poultry, lean cuts of meats, vegetables, and fruits.

Steaming

What it is and why it is healthy: Steaming involves cooking food by covering or enclosing it and then surrounding with steam. Steaming can be done either in the oven by wrapping food in foil or parchment packets, or on the stovetop using a steamer basket that sits above a pot of boiling water. Steaming cooks and seals in flavor, eliminating the need for added fats, and it is also one of the best cooking techniques for retaining nutrients.

What it is good for: Fish fillets, chicken breasts, shellfish, asparagus, green beans, leeks, and cruciferous vegetables, such as broccoli and cauliflower.

9 TIPS FOR EATING HEALTHFULLY ON A BUDGET

1. **Shop from a list:** A well-planned grocery list will keep you from buying unnecessary foods and lessen the chances of impulse buying.

2. **Use coupons and shop sales:** If you check the manufacturer's website of your favorite products, you can usually find online coupons that you can print.

3. **Look at unit prices:** The small stickers on the shelves tell you the price and also the unit price, which is how much the items cost per ounce, per pound, or for a standard number. Looking at the unit price is a quick and easy way to determine which brand is the best value.

4. **Incorporate more plant-based meals:** DASH recommends incorporating beans and legumes four or five times a week. A nutritional powerhouse of a food, beans and legumes are also very inexpensive and can serve as the foundation for several meatless meals each week.

5. **Buy in bulk:** Buying in bulk can save you a lot of money, let you try out new foods before purchasing in larger volumes, and allow you to cheaply add variety to your diet. Bulk foods generally keep for a long time; just store them in airtight containers.

6. **Buy in season:** Local produce is usually cheaper and higher in nutrients and flavor because it is picked at its peak. Stock up when your favorites are in season and freeze the excess.

7. **Buy frozen fruits and vegetables:** Contrary to what most people think, frozen fruits and vegetables are often *more* nutritious than their fresh counterparts. Fruits and vegetables are usually frozen within hours of being picked, which means they are packaged at their nutritional peak.

8. **Buy multiuse foods:** When you make your grocery list, think about the foods that you use in multiple recipes. For example, a large container of plain Greek yogurt is cheaper than individual containers and can be used in smoothies, in place of sour cream, to make sauces, and as a cereal topper.

9. **Be flexible:** Be willing to tweak your menu based on availability and last-minute sales. If your store happens to be out of some of your ingredients, don't scrap your whole menu and reach for processed foods. Instead, challenge yourself to modify your list/meal plan right there at the store. Some of the best meals come as a result of improvisation.

Broiling or Grilling

What it is and why it is healthy: Broiling and grilling both cook foods quickly by exposing them to direct heat; in the case of grilling, the heat comes from below, and with broiling, the heat comes from above. Both methods require the use of little (if any) added fats.

What it is good for: Broiling is good for tender cuts of meats, while grilling can be used for meats, vegetables, and fruits.

Poaching

What it is and why it is healthy: Poaching involves gently simmering food in water or a flavorful liquid like stock, wine, vinegar, or juice. Poaching doesn't require the use of fats or oils.

What it is good for: Chicken, fish, stone fruits, pears, and apples.

Meal Plan and Prep Like a Pro

You may have heard the popular adage attributed to Benjamin Franklin, "Failing to plan is planning to fail." Simple and to the point, this statement is applicable to so many areas of life, including meal planning. Meal planning doesn't have to be a time-consuming, laborious task that you dread each week. It can be done in 30 minutes or less. Good meal planning will save you time, money, and stress, and will make it so much easier to reach your health and weight-loss goals.

Some people like to use meal planning apps, templates, calendars, kitchen chalkboards or whiteboards, or are old-fashioned like me and simply use pen and paper. There's really no one best way to meal plan. The most important thing is simply to do it. After you read through this section, decide how you will meal plan. Dive right in and stick with your chosen method for a month or so. Once you have a chance to discover what works and doesn't work for you, then you can tweak your method as needed. Meal planning really boils down to four main tasks: choosing what you will cook, figuring out what ingredients you need, shopping for ingredients, and doing prep work for the week. The following list provides some additional tips and guidance to help you get started:

1. **SET ASIDE TIME TO MEAL PLAN** Sounds obvious, but unless you purposely carve out 20 to 30 minutes in your schedule each week to think calmly and plan, you probably won't do it. If Saturday is the day you shop, set aside time Friday night to get organized, then shop Saturday morning and do your prepping on Sunday.

2. **LOOK AT YOUR SCHEDULE FOR THE WEEK AND DECIDE HOW MANY MEALS YOU ARE GOING TO PREPARE** Do you have to work late on Thursday? Do the kids have a recital Wednesday night? List the exact number of meals you will need to prepare for the week including

breakfast, lunch, dinner, and snacks. Don't overwhelm yourself or set a lofty goal of cooking a meal from scratch seven days a week. Instead choose maybe three or four dinner recipes and factor in whether you can use the leftovers for lunches or another dinner on those busy nights. One other thing I personally do is have at least two "go-to" meals in my back pocket for those days/nights when everything goes wrong. Go-to meals are simply meals that you can put together quickly and always have the ingredients on hand. For example, if you always have eggs, frozen vegetables, and instant brown rice on hand, then in a pinch you could quickly prepare a nutritious stir-fry—a much healthier option than going to the drive-through, and almost the same amount of time required to get the meal on the table.

3. **DO A QUICK PANTRY/REFRIGERATOR/FREEZER INVENTORY** Are there foods that need to be used up? Do you have a large quantity of something, like a five-pound bag of carrots? Make a list of these items and see if you can incorporate recipes using these ingredients and list these recipes earlier in the week.

4. **GATHER YOUR RECIPES** Foster healthy habits by involving your family in recipe selection. Encourage them to try new foods. Keep things simple and make double portions when you can so that leftovers can be used for lunches or after-school snacks. As part of your DASH lifestyle, incorporate one or two meatless

meals each week and make "meatless Mondays" a new family tradition.

5. **PREPARE YOUR SHOPPING LIST** Make a list of the ingredients you need for the week making note of the foods you already have on hand. Remember to include what you need for breakfasts and snacks.

Prepping for the Week

Before you do your food prepping, be certain you have an arsenal of various sizes of storage containers with locking lids. Glass and stainless steel make good choices, and if you are going to use plastic, make sure it is BPA-free. Next take a look at your menu for the week and list out the foods that can be prepped in advance. For example, you could wash, chop, and prepare most of your vegetables for the week, prepare a week's worth of overnight oats, cook a big batch of whole grains, grill chicken breasts, cook lentils, portion out nuts for snacks, and boil eggs. Stack your containers in the refrigerator for easy access, or freeze perishables in recipe-ready portions. Lastly, consider labeling your containers with the day of the week and the meal each corresponds to. If you are freezing food, be sure to add the date you prepared it or its expiration date. If you are anything like me, taking time to plan, shop, and prep makes me feel so much calmer during the week, simply by knowing I have one less decision to make to answer the question: "What's for dinner?"

The DASH Weight-Loss Meal and Exercise Plans

Now that you have learned the features of the DASH diet, picked up some weight-loss tips, and know how to meal plan and prep like a pro, you are ready to transition to the DASH eating style. I have designed the following 1,600-calorie meal plans using recipes from this book so that you can jump right in without having to do any planning. Each week includes seven full days of meals and snacks with the calorie and nutrient totals listed so you can easily swap things out based on your personal preferences and individual calorie needs. The menu is high in fiber, keeps sodium in check, and emphasizes foods that are rich in potassium, magnesium, and calcium. While each day is designed to meet the daily food group recommendations of DASH, remember that on some days, you may eat a little more or less of a particular food group, which is fine. The goal is to meet the recommendations over the course of a few days or the week while still allowing flexibility in your choices, and for you to eat according to your hunger and fullness cues.

The calorie level of 1,600 is appropriate for most sedentary women over the age of 50, physically active women over the age of 50 who want to lose weight, and younger active women wanting to lose weight. An average male needs around 2,500 calories to maintain weight, and 2,000 to lose 1 pound per week. However, these numbers depend on a number of factors as discussed previously. These include age, height, current weight, activity levels, metabolic health, and others. If you did not calculate your daily calorie needs and target calories for weight loss as discussed earlier, take a moment now to do that (see Calculating Energy Needs, page 26). The National Institutes of Health offers a highly accurate and easy-to-use Body Weight Planner, an online tool that's automated to help you set your personal calorie and physical activity targets to meet your weight loss and management goals. The tool is available at https://www.niddk.nih.gov/bwp.

If you find your calorie goal for weight loss is higher than 1,600 calories, you can simply increase portion sizes of meals or snacks, add an additional snack, or add an extra serving of whole grain, protein,

vegetables, fruits, nuts, legumes, or healthy fats. "Essentials of Weight Loss" includes a list of ten snacks with around 150 calories each (see page 25), and each day of the plan has a listing of suggested snacks to be incorporated morning, afternoon, and evening, based on your hunger level and time between meals. Including nutritious, balanced snacks between meals prevents you from becoming overly hungry, which can lead to overeating at your next meal. Snacks also help to keep your energy up, blood sugar steady, and improve concentration. As a general guideline, try not to go more than five hours between meals so that you stay fueled for your day.

There are four weeks of meal plans for you to use to begin losing weight, each providing approximately 1,600 calories per day and meeting the recommendations of DASH. All recipes indicate serving sizes, so adjust accordingly based on the number of people in your household. Keep in mind that you may want to halve recipes or double them and freeze extras for leftovers. Each day will include a listing of suggested snacks as well. It is always best to let hunger be your guide, but have the snacks as needed throughout the day or with meals. The daily nutritional analysis includes all listed daily snacks.

The menus are designed to be simple to use and incorporate recipes that are quick to prepare. Each week includes a shopping list of all of the ingredients you will need for the week, but you will want to scan the recipes and check your pantry to avoid purchasing items you don't need. Plan on setting aside time on Saturday or Sunday to do your shopping and prepping for the week. Do as much food prep for the week as you can on the weekend so that your meals are ready to go during the week.

To make things easier to start and to cut down on preparation time, where possible, leftovers will be repurposed as lunches or as meals later in the week, and not all meals or snacks will require recipes. It helps to start slowly with meal planning, prep, and cooking to prevent you from feeling overwhelmed or burned out. You can also feel free to swap out recipes and foods depending on your personal preference—just try to choose recipes with a similar calorie count and aim to meet the DASH food group recommendations over the course of several days or the week as opposed to each day. The menus might be higher in fiber than you are used to, so remember to drink plenty of water or no-calorie beverages throughout the day. Full of fresh, whole foods, with lots of volume, each meal should leave you feeling energized and comfortably satisfied.

DASH Eating Plan: Number of Servings for a 1,600 calorie diet

FOOD GROUP	NUMBER OF SERVINGS
Grains	6
Vegetables	3 to 4
Fruits	4
Fat-free or low-fat dairy products	2 to 3
Lean meats, poultry, and fish	3 to 4 or less
Nuts, seeds, and legumes	3 to 4 per week
Fats and oils	2
Sweets and added sugars	3 or less per week
Maximum sodium per day	≤ 2,300 mg
Potassium	≥ 3,000 mg
Fiber	≥ 28 g

Progress, Not Perfection

Start slowly, and don't stress out if on some days, you stray from the plan. Change takes time, and you are aiming for progress, not perfection. Focus on the big picture—a healthy, sustainable lifestyle—and take one day at a time, celebrating each success, big and small. Also keep in mind: There is never a "perfect" time to start a lifestyle change like this. You may never feel *completely* ready to begin—and that's okay. Think about what's reasonable or realistic for you right now. Once you have completed the initial four weeks, use the template provided to sketch out your own plan using a combination of the recipes you have enjoyed the most, along with other recipes from the book or your own personal creations. Enjoy learning about and cooking new foods, experiencing new flavors, and relishing in the joy of doing something good for yourself. I always feel a sense of accomplishment when I immerse myself in cooking and prepare wholesome meals that feed my body, mind, and soul, and I hope you will, too.

WEEK ONE	SUNDAY	MEATLESS MONDAY	TUESDAY
Breakfast	• **Quick Skillet Sweet Potato and Black Bean Hash (page 83)** • ¼ medium avocado	• **Creamy Peach Quinoa (page 81)** • 1 cup fat-free milk	**Apple-Pistachio Overnight Oats (page 77)**
Morning Snack	Choose from list	Choose from list	Choose from list
Lunch	**Farmers' Market Chickpea Salad (page 108)**	• **Leftover Quick Skillet Sweet Potato and Black Bean Hash (page 83)** • 1 slice whole-grain bread and 2 tablespoons avocado	• **Leftover Creamy Cauliflower Butternut Squash Mac and Cheese (page 132)** • Salad: 2 cups spinach with 1 teaspoon extra-virgin olive oil
Afternoon Snack	Choose from list	Choose from list	Choose from list
Dinner	• **Roasted Cajun Blackened Salmon with Asparagus (page 163)** • ¾ cup brown rice • Salad: 2 cups spinach, 1 large tomato, and vinaigrette (made with ½ tablespoon extra-virgin olive oil)	• **Creamy Cauliflower Butternut Squash Mac and Cheese (page 132)** • Salad: 2 cups baby spinach and ½ tablespoon extra-virgin olive oil	• **Haddock Tacos with Cabbage Slaw (page 167)** • 1 cup steamed broccoli with 1 teaspoon extra-virgin olive oil
Evening Snack	Choose from list	Choose from list	Choose from list
Suggested Snacks	• 4-ounce container low-fat plain yogurt • 1 ounce low-fat cheese • 1 large banana • 1 orange	• One 100-calorie Greek yogurt • 1 medium apple • 1 low-fat string cheese • **1 Fudgy Chocolate Black Bean Cookie (page 228)**	• 1 medium banana • 1 cup fat-free milk • **1 Single-Serve Cherry-Vanilla Cupcake (page 231)**
Nutritional Analysis for the Day	Calories 1,650, Total fat: 55 g, Saturated fat: 10 g, Cholesterol: 88 mg, Sodium: 631 mg, Potassium: 4,051 mg, Total carbohydrates: 216 g, Fiber: 51 g, Sugars: 59 g, Protein: 93 g	Calories: 1,608, Total fat: 41 g, Saturated fat: 8 g, Cholesterol: 41 mg, Sodium: 1,243 mg, Potassium: 3,059 mg, Total carbohydrates: 235 g, Fiber: 52 g, Sugars: 16 g, Protein: 89 g	Calories: 1,658, Total fat: 48 g, Saturated fat: 8 g, Cholesterol: 115 mg, Sodium: 1,369 mg, Potassium: 3,251 mg, Total carbohydrates: 216 g, Fiber: 45 g, Sugars: 75 g, Protein: 108 g

WEDNESDAY	THURSDAY	FRIDAY	SATURDAY
• **Leftover Creamy Peach Quinoa (page 81)** • ½ cup low-fat vanilla yogurt	**Chocolate-Cherry Smoothie Bowl (page 73)**	• **Leftover Creamy Peach Quinoa (page 81)** • ½ cup 1% cottage cheese	• **2-Minute Egg and Vegetable Breakfast Mug (page 86)** • 1 slice whole-grain bread • ½ medium tomato, sliced • ¼ cup avocado slices
Choose from list	Choose from list	Choose from list	Choose from list
• **Leftover Haddock Tacos with Cabbage Slaw (page 167)** • 1 cup steamed zucchini	• **Leftover Oatmeal-Crusted Chicken Tenders (page 159)** • **Leftover Herbed Cauliflower and Broccoli Rice (page 211)**	• **Leftover Slow Cooker Rosemary Pork and Root Vegetables (page 177)** • 1 orange	**Leftover Lemongrass Coconut Curry Chicken (page 156)**
Choose from list	Choose from list	Choose from list	Choose from list
• **Oatmeal-Crusted Chicken Tenders (page 159)** • **Herbed Cauliflower and Broccoli Rice (page 211)** • Salad: 2 cups baby spinach and ½ tablespoon extra-virgin olive oil	• **Slow Cooker Rosemary Pork and Root Vegetables (page 177)** • Salad: 2 cups baby spinach and ½ tablespoon extra-virgin olive oil	• **Lemongrass Coconut Curry Chicken (page 156)** • Salad: 2 cups spinach, 1 large tomato, and vinaigrette (made with ½ tablespoon extra-virgin olive oil)	• **Open-Faced Veggie-Packed Beef Burger (page 186)** served on a whole-grain hamburger bun (around 130 calories) • ½ cup spinach and ½ tomato • **Crispy Baked Zucchini Fries (page 221)**
Choose from list	Choose from list	Choose from list	Choose from list
• 1 large banana • ½ cup low-fat vanilla yogurt • 1 orange • 1 ounce almonds • **1 Fudgy Chocolate Black Bean Cookie (page 228)**	• 1 cup fat-free milk • ¼ cup dried apricots • 1 ounce pistachios • 1 orange	• 1 cup fat-free milk • 1 large banana • 1 ounce low-fat cheese • 2 cups air-popped popcorn	• 1 cup low-fat plain yogurt • 1 orange • 1 large banana • **1 Fudgy Chocolate Black Bean Cookie (page 228)**
Calories: 1,639, Total fat: 62 g, Saturated fat: 10 g, Cholesterol: 171 mg, Sodium: 1,336 mg, Potassium: 3,306 mg, Total carbohydrates: 178 g, Fiber: 32 g, Sugars: 66 g, Protein: 106 g	Calories: 1,620, Total fat: 61 g, Saturated fat: 10 g, Cholesterol: 22 mg, Sodium: 1,233 mg, Potassium: 4,760 mg, Total carbohydrates: 165 g, Fiber: 32 g, Sugars: 90 g, Protein: 125 g	Calories: 1,632, Total fat: 39 g, Saturated fat: 11 g, Cholesterol: 221 mg, Sodium: 1,296 mg, Potassium: 3,766 mg, Total carbohydrates: 202 g, Fiber: 28 g, Sugars: 73 g, Protein: 129 g	Calories: 1,639, Total fat: 47 g, Saturated fat: 15 g, Cholesterol: 546 mg, Sodium: 1,293 mg, Potassium: 3,250 mg, Total carbohydrates: 210 g, Fiber: 35 g, Sugars: 71 g, Protein: 110 g

WEEK TWO

	SUNDAY	MEATLESS MONDAY	TUESDAY
Breakfast	**Apple-Pistachio Overnight Oats (page 77)**	• **Apricot-Banana Breakfast Barley (page 80)** • ½ cup low-fat plain yogurt	**Green Apple Pie Protein Smoothie (page 72)**
Morning Snack	Choose from list	Choose from list	Choose from list
Lunch	**Curried Roasted Cauliflower and Lentil Salad (page 109)**	**Leftover Curried Roasted Cauliflower and Lentil Salad (page 109)**	**Leftover Bean Pasta with Arugula Avocado Walnut Pesto (page 135)**
Afternoon Snack	Choose from list	Choose from list	Choose from list
Dinner	• **Easy Scallop Quinoa Paella (page 172)** • Salad: 2 cups spinach, 1 teaspoon extra-virgin olive oil	**Bean Pasta with Arugula Avocado Walnut Pesto (page 135)**	• **Chicken and Beet Soup (page 122)** • **Avocado Tomato Ricotta Toast (page 84)**
Evening Snack	Choose from list	Choose from list	Choose from list
Suggested Snacks	• **1 High-Protein Apple Carrot Hemp Muffin (page 89)** • 1 cup fat-free milk • 1 large banana	• **1 High-Protein Apple Carrot Hemp Muffin (page 89)** • **1 Single-Serve Cherry-Vanilla Cupcake (page 231)** • ½ cup low-fat plain yogurt • 1 medium orange	• **1 High-Protein Apple Carrot Hemp Muffin (page 89)** • 2 oranges • 1 cup fat-free milk
Nutritional Analysis for the Day	Calories: 1,623, Total fat: 44 g, Saturated fat: 3 g, Cholesterol: 47 mg, Sodium: 906 mg, Potassium: 4,062 mg, Total carbohydrates: 238 g, Fiber: 58 g, Sugars: 79 g, Protein: 93 g	Calories: 1,631, Total fat: 52g, Saturated fat: 8 g, Cholesterol: 18 mg, Sodium: 916 mg, Potassium: 3,276 mg, Total carbohydrates: 235 g, Fiber: 58 g, Sugars: 71 g, Protein: 85 g	Calories: 1,638, Total fat: 55 g, Saturated fat: 7 g, Cholesterol: 85 mg, Sodium: 1,331 mg, Potassium: 3,879 mg, Total carbohydrates: 216 g, Fiber: 48 g, Sugars: 88 g, Protein: 101 g

WEDNESDAY	THURSDAY	FRIDAY	SATURDAY
• **Leftover Apricot-Banana Breakfast Barley (page 80)** • ½ cup low-fat plain yogurt	**Raspberry Mango Turmeric Overnight Oats (page 77)**	• **Leftover Apricot-Banana Breakfast Barley (page 80)** • ½ cup low-fat plain yogurt	• **2 High-Protein Apple Carrot Hemp Muffins (page 89)** • 2 teaspoons peanut butter • 1 cup low-fat milk
Choose from list	Choose from list	Choose from list	Choose from list
• **Leftover Chicken and Beet Soup (page 122)** • **Avocado Tomato Ricotta Toast (page 84)**	**Leftover Bean, Squash, and Tomato Stew (page 116)**	• **Leftover Sweet and Savory Apple-Cinnamon Baked Pork Chops (page 179)** • 1 small baked sweet potato • 1 cup steamed zucchini, 1 teaspoon extra-virgin olive oil	• **Leftover Roasted Salmon, Spinach, and Butternut Squash Salad (page 92)** • 1 cup steamed broccoli
Choose from list	Choose from list	Choose from list	Choose from list
Bean, Squash, and Tomato Stew (page 116)	• **Sweet and Savory Apple-Cinnamon Baked Pork Chops (page 179)** • 1 medium baked sweet potato • 1 cup steamed zucchini, 1 teaspoon extra-virgin olive oil	• **Roasted Salmon, Spinach, and Butternut Squash Salad (page 92)** • 1 thin slice whole-grain bread	• **Steak with Red Onions, Peppers, and Mushrooms (page 185)** • ½ cup cooked brown rice • 1 cup steamed zucchini, 1 teaspoon extra-virgin olive oil
Choose from list	Choose from list	Choose from list	Choose from list
• **1 High-Protein Apple Carrot Hemp Muffin (page 89)** • 1 cup diced cantaloupe • 1 cup fat-free milk	• **1 High-Protein Apple Carrot Hemp Muffin (page 89)** • 1 cup diced cantaloupe • 1 cup fat-free milk	• **1 High-Protein Apple Carrot Hemp Muffin (page 89)** • ½ cup low-fat plain yogurt • 2 kiwifruits	• 1 orange • ¼ cup pistachios • 1 medium banana • 1½ ounces low-fat hard cheese (Swiss, cheddar, etc.)
Calories: 1,611, Total fat: 47 g, Saturated fat: 8 g, Cholesterol: 89 g, Sodium: 1,214 mg, Potassium: 4,637 mg, Total carbohydrates: 234 g, Fiber: 48 g, Sugars: 88 g, Protein: 89 g	Calories: 1,638, Total fat: 48 g, Saturated fat: 8 g, Cholesterol: 76 mg, Sodium: 634 mg, Potassium: 4,508 mg, Total carbohydrates: 238 g, Fiber: 50 g, Sugars: 98 g, Protein: 83 g	Calories: 1,616, Total fat: 51 g, Saturated fat: 11 g, Cholesterol: 209 mg, Sodium: 851 mg, Potassium: 3,993 mg, Total carbohydrates: 205 g, Fiber: 37 g, Sugars: 77 g, Protein: 99 g	Calories: 1,619, Total fat: 64 g, Saturated fat: 11 g, Cholesterol: 207 mg, Sodium: 1,023 mg, Potassium: 3,833 mg, Total carbohydrates: 170 g, Fiber: 34 g, Sugars: 67 g, Protein: 108 g

WEEK THREE	SUNDAY	MEATLESS MONDAY	TUESDAY
Breakfast	**Banana-Almond Pancakes for One (page 87)**	**Avocado Tomato Ricotta Toast (page 84)**	• **Strawberry Orange Beet Smoothie (page 74)** • **Strawberry Almond Ricotta Toast (page 84)**
Morning Snack	Choose from list	Choose from list	Choose from list
Lunch	**Barley and Roasted Brussels Sprouts with Fresh Herbs and Ricotta (page 94)**	**Leftover Barley and Roasted Brussels Sprouts with Fresh Herbs and Ricotta (page 94)**	• **Leftover Two-Potato Cauliflower Soup (page 125)** • **Leftover Butternut Squash and Sage Portobello Mushroom Pizzas (page 212)**
Afternoon Snack	Choose from list	Choose from list	Choose from list
Dinner	• **Lemon-Garlic Tilapia with Roasted Vegetables and Arugula (page 171)** • **Lightened-Up Creamed Corn (page 216)**	• **Two-Potato Cauliflower Soup (page 125)** • **Butternut Squash and Sage Portobello Mushroom Pizzas (page 212)**	• **One-Pot Shrimp Pasta Primavera (page 166)** • Salad: 2 cups spinach, 1 medium tomato, 1 teaspoon extra-virgin olive oil
Evening Snack	Choose from list	Choose from list	Choose from list
Suggested Snacks	• 1 orange • 1 cup fat-free milk • 1 (5.3-ounce) container nonfat (0%) Greek yogurt • 1 ounce almonds • 1 cup strawberry halves	• 1 cup low-fat (2%) plain Greek yogurt • 1 orange • 1 medium banana • **Cheesy Baked Kale Chips (page 209)**	• 1 cup fat-free milk • 1 large banana • **Cheesy Baked Kale Chips (page 209)**
Nutritional Analysis for the Day	Calories: 1,627, Total fat: 59 g, Saturated fat: 13 g, Cholesterol: 450 mg, Sodium: 838 mg, Potassium: 4,184 mg, Total carbohydrates: 198 g, Fiber: 40 g, Sugars: 76 g, Protein: 98 g	Calories: 1,609, Total fat: 59 g, Saturated fat: 14 g, Cholesterol: 66 mg, Sodium: 1,040 mg, Potassium: 4,459 mg, Total carbohydrates: 223 g, Fiber: 46 g, Sugars: 71 g, Protein: 79 g	Calories: 1,616, Total fat: 49 g, Saturated fat: 9 g, Cholesterol: 161 mg, Sodium: 1,376 mg, Potassium: 4,497 mg, Total carbohydrates: 225 g, Fiber: 43 g, Sugars: 81 g, Protein: 86 g

WEDNESDAY	THURSDAY	FRIDAY	SATURDAY
Pumpkin-Flax Overnight Oats (page 77)	• **Blueberry-Walnut Steel-Cut Oats (page 76)** • ½ cup low-fat plain yogurt	**Green Apple Pie Protein Smoothie (page 72)**	• **Leftover Blueberry-Walnut Steel-Cut Oats (page 76)** • ½ cup low fat plain yogurt
Choose from list	Choose from list	Choose from list	Choose from list
Leftover One-Pot Shrimp Pasta Primavera (page 166)	• **Leftover Crispy Walnut Chicken with Steamed Broccoli (page 153)** • 1 cup baby carrots	• **Leftover Restaurant-Style Pork Fajitas (page 181)** • ½ cup black beans	**Leftover Lentil Sloppy Joes (page 138)** served on whole-grain hamburger bun with ½ medium avocado
Choose from list	Choose from list	Choose from list	Choose from list
• **Crispy Walnut Chicken with Steamed Broccoli (page 153)** • Salad; 2 cups spinach, 1 medium tomato, ½ avocado, 1 teaspoon extra-virgin olive oil	• **Restaurant-Style Pork Fajitas (page 181)** • 1 cup warmed black beans • Salad: 2 cups spinach, 1 medium tomato, 1 teaspoon extra-virgin olive oil	**Lentil Sloppy Joes (page 138)** served on whole-grain hamburger bun with ½ medium avocado, 1 cup steamed zucchini	• **Easy Skillet Swiss Steak (page 184)** • 1 small baked sweet potato • 1 cup steamed broccoli with 2 teaspoons extra-virgin olive oil
Choose from list	Choose from list	Choose from list	Choose from list
• 1 orange • 1 large banana • 1 cup low-fat plain yogurt • 1 thin slice whole-grain bread with 1 tablespoon nut butter	• ½ cup low-fat plain yogurt • 1½ ounces low-fat hard cheese • 1 cup diced cantaloupe • 1 orange	• 1 cup baby carrots • 1 large banana • 1 cup fat-free milk • 1 ounce low-fat hard cheese	• ½ cup low-fat plain yogurt • 1 cup strawberry halves • 1 ounce pistachios • 1 orange
Calories: 1,612, Total fat: 62 g, Saturated fat: 9 g, Cholesterol: 190 mg, Sodium: 1,052 mg, Potassium: 3,113 mg, Total carbohydrates: 191 g, Fiber: 39 g, Sugars: 64 g, Protein: 99 g	Calories: 1,602, Total fat: 54 g, Saturated fat: 10 g, Cholesterol: 147 mg, Sodium: 1,130 mg, Potassium: 4,154 mg, Total carbohydrates: 183 g, Fiber: 46 g, Sugars: 60 g, Protein: 113 g	Calories: 1,618, Total fat: 39 g, Saturated fat: 7 g, Cholesterol: 83 mg, Sodium: 1,532 mg, Potassium: 4,950 mg, Total carbohydrates: 236 g, Fiber: 57 g, Sugars: 74 g, Protein: 97 g	Calories: 1,635, Total fat: 64 g, Saturated fat: 14 g, Cholesterol: 78 mg, Sodium: 1,335 mg, Potassium: 3,414 mg, Total carbohydrates: 201 g, Fiber: 45 g, Sugars: 61 g, Protein: 80 g

WEEK FOUR	SUNDAY	MEATLESS MONDAY	TUESDAY
Breakfast	Chocolate-Cherry Smoothie Bowl (page 73)	Raspberry Mango Turmeric Overnight Oats (page 77)	• 2 Strawberry-Banana Protein Muffins (page 230) • 1 cup low-fat plain yogurt
Morning Snack	Choose from list	Choose from list	Choose from list
Lunch	• Barley Soup with Asparagus and Mushrooms (page 121) • Salad: 1 cup baby greens and ½ small avocado	• Leftover Barley Soup with Asparagus and Mushrooms (page 121) • Salad: 1 cup baby greens and ½ small avocado	• Leftover Aromatic Chickpea Stew (page 124) • 1 thin slice whole-grain bread with ½ small avocado
Afternoon Snack	Choose from list	Choose from list	Choose from list
Dinner	• Lemon-Ginger Tilapia with Roasted Vegetables and Arugula (page 171) • Salad: 1 cup spinach, ½ medium tomato, ½ tablespoon extra-virgin olive oil	• Aromatic Chickpea Stew (page 124) • 1 thin slice whole-grain bread with ½ small avocado	• Chicken and Vegetable Stir-Fry (page 152) • ½ cup brown rice • Salad: 2 cups spinach, ½ medium tomato, ½ tablespoon extra-virgin olive oil
Evening Snack	Choose from list	Choose from list	Choose from list
Suggested Snacks	• 1 Strawberry-Banana Protein Muffin (page 230) • 1 orange • 1 cup fat-free milk	• 1 Strawberry-Banana Protein Muffin (page 230) • 1 medium banana with 1 tablespoon peanut butter • 1 (5.3-ounce) container nonfat (0%) Greek yogurt	• 2 oranges • 1 ounce almonds • 1 (5.3-ounce) container nonfat (0%) Greek yogurt
Nutritional Analysis for the Day	Calories: 1,635, Total fat: 50 g, Saturated fat: 7 g, Cholesterol: 88 mg, Sodium: 737 mg, Potassium: 4,681 mg, Total carbohydrates: 233 g, Fiber: 47 g, Sugars: 77 g, Protein: 86 g	Calories: 1,642, Total fat: 46 g, Saturated fat: 4 g, Cholesterol: 21 mg, Sodium: 704 mg, Potassium: 4,150 mg, Total carbohydrates: 253 g, Fiber: 59 g, Sugars: 70 g, Protein: 82 g	Calories: 1,627, Total fat: 54 g, Saturated fat: 6 g, Cholesterol: 102 mg, Sodium: 944 mg, Potassium: 4,122 mg, Total carbohydrates: 200 g, Fiber: 43 g, Sugars: 76 g, Protein: 101 g

WEDNESDAY	THURSDAY	FRIDAY	SATURDAY
Green Apple Pie Protein Smoothie (page 72)	• **2 Strawberry-Banana Protein Muffins (page 230)** • 1 cup low-fat plain yogurt	Avocado Tomato Ricotta Toast (page 84)	Banana-Almond Pancakes for One (page 87)
Choose from list	Choose from list	Choose from list	Choose from list
• **Leftover Chicken and Vegetable Stir-Fry (page 152)** • ½ cup brown rice	• **Leftover Beef Tenderloin with Chickpeas and Artichoke Hearts (page 188)** • 1 small sweet potato with 2 tablespoons shredded low-fat cheese	Simple Shrimp Salad for Two with Ginger Vinaigrette (page 98)	• **Grilled Turkey and Avocado Salad (page 104)** • 1 cup steamed broccoli with 1 teaspoon extra-virgin olive oil
Choose from list	Choose from list	Choose from list	Choose from list
• **Beef Tenderloin with Chickpeas and Artichoke Hearts (page 188)** • 1 small sweet potato with 2 tablespoons shredded low-fat cheese • Salad: 2 cups spinach, ½ medium tomato, 1 teaspoon extra-virgin olive oil	• **Orange-Thyme Salmon and Summer Squash in a Packet (page 164)** • Salad: 2 cups spinach, ½ medium tomato, ½ tablespoon extra-virgin olive oil	Pistachio-Crusted Honey-Mustard Turkey Cutlets with Radicchio Slaw (page 155)	• **Lentil-Walnut Mushroom Tacos (page 139)** • 1 cup steamed broccoli with 1 teaspoon extra-virgin olive oil
Choose from list	Choose from list	Choose from list	Choose from list
• **1 Strawberry-Banana Protein Muffin (page 230)** with 1 tablespoon peanut butter • 1 orange • 1 (5.3-ounce) container nonfat (0%) Greek yogurt	• 1 cup raspberries • 1 ounce walnuts • 1 orange • 2 Hershey's Dark Chocolate Kisses	• **1 Strawberry-Banana Protein Muffin (page 230)** • 1 orange • 1 large banana • ½ cup low-fat plain yogurt	• **1 Strawberry-Banana Protein Muffin (page 230)** with 1 teaspoon peanut butter • 1 cup low-fat plain yogurt • 1 cup raspberries
Calories: 1,610, Total fat: 43 g, Saturated fat: 7 g, Cholesterol: 139 mg, Sodium: 1,024 mg, Potassium: 4,093 mg, Total carbohydrates: 195 g, Fiber: 42 g, Sugars: 58 g, Protein: 119 g	Calories: 1,625, Total fat: 60 g, Saturated fat: 12 g, Cholesterol: 186 mg, Sodium: 1,204 mg, Potassium: 4,091 mg, Total carbohydrates: 172 g, Fiber: 44 g, Sugars: 68 g, Protein: 114 g	Calories: 1,617, Total fat: 65 g, Saturated fat: 11 g, Cholesterol: 393 mg, Sodium: 1,617 mg, Potassium: 3,058 mg, Total carbohydrates: 164 g, Fiber: 33 g, Sugars: 76 g, Protein: 103 g	Calories: 1,623, Total fat: 80 g, Saturated fat: 13 g, Cholesterol: 473 mg, Sodium: 712 mg, Potassium: 4,385 mg, Total carbohydrates: 151 g, Fiber: 50 g, Sugars: 64 g, Protein: 99 g

The Exercise Plan

In addition to diet, physical activity is an integral part of a weight-loss plan and a healthy, sustainable lifestyle. And just like making dietary changes, there is no one perfect time to start; plus, changing your level of fitness takes time, so be patient and focus on your long-term goals and on progress, not perfection.

A balanced fitness plan should include cardiovascular exercise, strength training, and stretching/flexibility exercises. But before jumping in, it is imperative to acknowledge your current level of fitness and consult a physician for approval if necessary. The workouts in this chapter offer modifications, progression guidance, and explanation.

One of the first things you should learn is what is considered "moderate" physical activity, and what it feels like. The Borg Rating of Perceived Exertion (RPE) is a way of measuring physical activity level based on the sensations you experience during exercise, including increased heart rate, increased sweating, increased breathing rate, and muscle fatigue.[1] RPE has been found to correlate well with actual heart rate during physical activity, making it a good tool to self-monitor how hard you are working so that you can adjust the intensity of the activity as needed. The standard scale that you will often see uses a range of 0 to 20; however, I prefer a simpler version ranging from 0 to 10, which is easier to use and remember. When you are exercising, ask yourself how you feel, how hard you are working, and how much sweat effort you feel like you are expending. How easily you can talk while exercising factors into this scale as well, and is an easy way to gauge effort.

In general, for moderate-intensity cardiovascular exercise, you want your RPE to be around a level 5 or 6 out of 10. For vigorous intensity exercise, aim for an RPE level of 7 to 8. Working out at level 10 is not recommended for most workouts. For longer, slower workouts, keep your RPE at level 5 or lower. At least 10 minutes of continuous physical activity is needed for it to be considered an exercise session. Thirty minutes of moderate physical activity 5 days per week, or a total of 2 hours 30 minutes per week is recommended. The following chart lists the ratings of perceived exertion on a 10-point scale:

RATINGS OF PERCEIVED EXERTION

0 – Nothing at all, sitting

0.5 – Just noticeable

1 – Very light

2 – Light, you could maintain this pace all day

3 – Still comfortable, breathing a bit harder

4 – Sweating a little, but can still talk effortlessly

5 – Just above comfortable, sweating more, can still talk easily

6 – Can still talk but slightly breathless

7 – Hard to talk, breathing heavy

8 – Hard effort, can only keep this pace for a short time, too breathless to talk

9 – Extremely hard effort

10 – Maximum exertion

Strength Training

Building muscle through the use of strength exercises is essential for boosting your metabolism and helping you to maintain strong bones. An effective routine will ideally work each of the major muscle groups in your body including chest, arms, back, abdominals, and legs (hamstrings, quadriceps, and glutes/buttocks). If you are a beginner, start with the basic total body circuit to build a strong foundation in all of your muscle groups. A body-weight circuit means you simply use the weight of your body for resistance without adding dumbbells or other types of resistance such as bands. If you have been working out for a while, use the intermediate/advanced circuit. In either case, always warm up with light cardiovascular exercise such as riding a stationary bike or walking at a moderate pace for 5 to 10 minutes. From the table (see page 66), choose at least one exercise per muscle group and complete 1 to 3 sets of 10 to 12 repetitions. For your chest, choose exercises including chest press, push-ups, or bench press; for your back: one-arm row, back extensions, lateral pulldown; for your shoulders: overhead press, lateral raises, front raises, upright rows; for your biceps: dumbbell bicep curls, resistance band curls, hammer curls; for your triceps: lying triceps extensions, seated triceps extensions, triceps dips, triceps kickbacks; for your lower body: squats, lunges, deadlifts, calf raises, step-ups; for your abdominals: planks, bicycles, ball crunches.

STRETCHING 101

Active stretches increase flexibility and are done without any external help. Stretches should be held for 10 to 15 seconds. Some examples include:

- Quadriceps stretch: Stand upright and stretch the front of your thigh by lifting your leg behind you and gently grasping your ankle and lifting upward. Hold for 10 to 15 seconds and release.

- Shoulder, chest, leg, and back stretch: Stand with feet wide, clasp hands behind you with palms together and arms extended. Bend forward from hips until back is parallel to floor as you raise arms up. Hold for 10 to 15 seconds and slowly rise to starting position.

- Hamstring stretch: Touch your toes by gently folding over until you reach a comfortable stretch, hold for 10 to 15 seconds and release.

- Hip stretch: Step one foot forward while gently dropping the opposite knee to the floor. Place your hands on the forward knee and hold for 10 to 15 seconds. Repeat on the opposite side.

The following simple 4-week plan incorporates cardiovascular exercise, strength exercises, and stretching, which you can incorporate into your lifestyle based on your work schedule and time commitments. The beginner plan does not require any equipment; however, as you get stronger, you might think about purchasing resistance bands, a set of dumbbells, or a kettlebell. The intermediate/advanced plan can be done using only body weight; however, depending on your weight- and fat-loss goals, using some type of resistance will make the workout more challenging, build your strength, and increase your benefits. The intensity of the workout should be moderate, around a level 5 or 6 of the RPE.

If something in the program doesn't meet your needs, figure out what is not working and simply swap out exercises and change it the next week. While following the 4-week workout routine may be effective, the best workouts are ones you enjoy. There are numerous workouts to choose from, so continue to experiment until you develop a healthy and enjoyable relationship with physical activity.

WEEK ONE	BEGINNER	INTERMEDIATE/ADVANCED
DAY 1	• Walk 15 to 20 minutes • Active stretches (see page 63)	• 30 to 60 minutes of moderate activity • Active stretches (see page 63)
DAY 2	• Walk 15 to 20 minutes • Active stretches • Body-weight circuit (see page 66)	• 30 to 60 minutes of moderate activity • Active stretches • Strength circuit (see page 66)
DAY 3	Rest day	Rest day
DAY 4	• Walk 15 to 20 minutes • Active stretches	• 30 to 60 minutes of moderate activity • Active stretches
DAY 5	• Walk 15 to 20 minutes • Active stretches • Body-weight circuit	• 30 to 60 minutes of moderate activity • Active stretches • Strength circuit
DAY 6	• Walk 15 to 20 minutes • Active stretches	• 30 to 60 minutes of moderate activity • Active stretches
DAY 7	Rest day	Rest day

Examples of Exercise Intensity

LIGHT-INTENSITY ACTIVITIES	MODERATE-INTENSITY ACTIVITIES	VIGOROUS-INTENSITY ACTIVITIES
• Washing dishes • Watching television • Walking at around 1.7 mph	• Walking at 3 to 3.4 mph • Bicycling at less than 10 mph • Water aerobics	• Race-walking, jogging, or running • Jumping rope • Swimming laps

WEEK TWO	BEGINNER	INTERMEDIATE/ADVANCED
DAY 1	• Walk 20 minutes • Active stretches	• 30 to 60 minutes of moderate activity • Active stretches
DAY 2	• Walk 20 minutes • Active stretches • Body-weight circuit	• 30 to 60 minutes of moderate activity • Active stretches • Strength circuit
DAY 3	Rest day	Rest day
DAY 4	• Walk 20 minutes • Active stretches	• 30 to 60 minutes of moderate activity • Active stretches
DAY 5	• Walk 20 minutes • Active stretches • Body-weight circuit	• 30 to 60 minutes of moderate activity • Active stretches • Strength circuit
DAY 6	• Walk 20 minutes • Active stretches	• 30 to 60 minutes of moderate activity • Active stretches
DAY 7	Rest day	Rest day

WEEK THREE	BEGINNER	INTERMEDIATE/ADVANCED
DAY 1	• Walk 25 to 30 minutes • Active stretches	• 45 to 60 minutes of moderate activity • Active stretches • Strength circuit
DAY 2	• Walk 25 to 30 minutes • Active stretches • Body-weight circuit	• 45 to 60 minutes of moderate activity • Active stretches
DAY 3	Rest day	Rest day
DAY 4	• Walk 25 to 30 minutes • Active stretches	• 45 to 60 minutes of moderate activity • Active stretches • Strength circuit
DAY 5	• Walk 25 to 30 minutes • Active stretches • Body-weight circuit	• 45 to 60 minutes of moderate activity • Active stretches
DAY 6	• Walk 25 to 30 minutes • Active stretches	• 45 to 60 minutes of moderate activity • Active stretches • Strength circuit
DAY 7	Rest day	Rest day

Body-Weight and Strength Circuits

The following chart illustrates two different circuits: a beginner circuit where no weights are used except the weight of your body, and a more advanced circuit, which uses a light set of dumbbells.

SAMPLE BEGINNER BODY-WEIGHT CIRCUIT EQUIPMENT NEEDED: NONE	SAMPLE INTERMEDIATE/ADVANCED STRENGTH CIRCUIT EQUIPMENT NEEDED: ONE SET OF LIGHT DUMBBELLS
• Wall squats (30 seconds, or as tolerated) • Wall push-ups (10 to 12 reps) • Lunges (5 per leg, 10 total) • Triceps dips (10 to 12 reps) • Bicycles (20) • Planks (30 seconds, or as tolerated) Rest and repeat for a total of 1 to 3 sets	• Squats (10 to 12 reps) holding light dumbbells • Lunges (5 per leg, 10 total) holding light dumbbells • Jumping jacks (20) • Push-ups (10 to 12 reps) • Lateral raises (10 to 12 reps) holding light dumbbells • Planks (30 seconds or as tolerated) • Triceps dips (10 to 12 reps) • Bicep curls (10 to 12 reps) using light dumbbells • High knees (20) • One-arm rows (5 per arm, 10 total) using light dumbbells • Bicycles (20) Rest and repeat for a total of 2 to 3 sets.

WEEK FOUR	BEGINNER	INTERMEDIATE/ADVANCED
DAY 1	• Walk 30 minutes • Active stretches	• 45 to 60 minutes of moderate activity • Active stretches • Strength circuit
DAY 2	• Walk 30 minutes • Active stretches • Body-weight circuit	• 45 to 60 minutes of moderate activity • Active stretches
DAY 3	Rest day	Rest day
DAY 4	• Walk 30 minutes • Active stretches	• 45 to 60 minutes of moderate activity • Active stretches • Strength circuit
DAY 5	• Walk 30 minutes • Active stretches • Body-weight circuit	• 45 to 60 minutes of moderate activity • Active stretches
DAY 6	• Walk 30 minutes • Active stretches	• 45 to 60 minutes of moderate activity • Active stretches • Strength circuit
DAY 7	Rest day	Rest day

The Recipes

In the following pages, you can take everything you've learned about the DASH diet and weight loss, and put it all into practice by applying those principles in the kitchen. I have created 100 delicious, creative, nutrient-dense, whole-food recipes that will appeal to the entire family. The recipes were purposely developed to be high in nutrients proven to support healthy blood pressure levels, lower cholesterol, and aid in weight management and weight loss. In particular, the recipes are high in potassium, calcium, magnesium, and fiber, and low in saturated fat and sodium. The use of sodium is minimal, so if you do not have sodium restrictions, feel free to use your judgment to increase the amount. However, keep in mind that just 1 teaspoon of salt contains your entire day's worth of sodium: 2,400 milligrams.

As a general rule, always read through a recipe completely before you begin so you know what to expect in terms of steps, preparation, and time. The recipes all have headnotes that describe the recipe, an estimated preparation time, cooking time, and approximate yield. At the end of each recipe, you will find tips with additional information related to the ingredients (selection, storage, other uses), substitutions for different diets, preparation methods, advice for storing leftovers, or nutrient content of ingredients. Lastly, each recipe has been tested in home kitchens and sampled by eager samplers in order to ensure they are tasty, reliable, and accurate.

Substitutions and Guides

Did you ever come home from the grocery store and forget several items that you had written on your list? I know I have! Luckily there are ways to work around this by choosing appropriate ingredient substitutions.

INGREDIENT	SUBSTITUTION
Juice of a fresh lemon or lime	2 tablespoons juice
Shallot	Minced onion plus a pinch of garlic powder or minced garlic
Kale	Spinach
Lemongrass	Lemon zest
Balsamic vinegar	Red wine vinegar
Flaxseed	Chia seed
Honey	Maple syrup
Basil	Oregano or thyme
Cilantro	Parsley
Cumin	Chili powder
Dill	Tarragon
Chili powder	Dash bottled hot sauce plus oregano and cumin
Ginger	Allspice, cinnamon, or nutmeg
Mint	Basil or marjoram
Coriander	Ground caraway seed or cumin

Note: For any herb, you can substitute 1 teaspoon dried herb for 1 tablespoon fresh herb (with some exceptions, i.e., rosemary)

Recipe Nutrition Information

Each recipe contains a listing of nutritional information including calories, total fat, saturated fat, cholesterol, sodium, potassium, total carbohydrates, fiber, sugars (this includes both natural and added), and protein. Nutritional values used in the calculations either come from the USDA Agricultural Research Service Nutrient Database or food manufacturers.

Due to variations in ingredients and measurements, keep in mind that nutrient calculations are estimates and values are approximations. Please use them as a guide only, until you become familiar with the amount of food that keeps you feeling full and satisfied. Once you have completed the 4-week meal plan, which includes a detailed nutrient breakdown, you should be able to let your appetite be your guide, and use the information as a reference point for moving forward with your DASH weight-loss and maintenance plan.

Grain and Bean Cooking Guide

BEAN OR GRAIN (1 CUP DRY)	WATER (CUPS)	COOK TIME (MINUTES)	YIELD (CUPS)
Lentils, brown	2¼	20 to 25	2¼
Lentils, green	2	20 to 25	2
Lentils, red or yellow	3	15 to 20	2 to 2½
Pearl barley	2½	40 to 50	3 to 3½
Quinoa	2	15 to 20	2¾
Rice, brown basmati	2½	35 to 40	3
Rice, brown, long-grain	2½	45 to 55	3
Rice, brown, short-grain	2 to 2½	45 to 55	3
Rice, brown, quick-cooking	1¼	10	2
Oat bran	2	5 to 7	2⅔
Rolled oats	2	10	2
Steel-cut oats	4	20 to 40	4

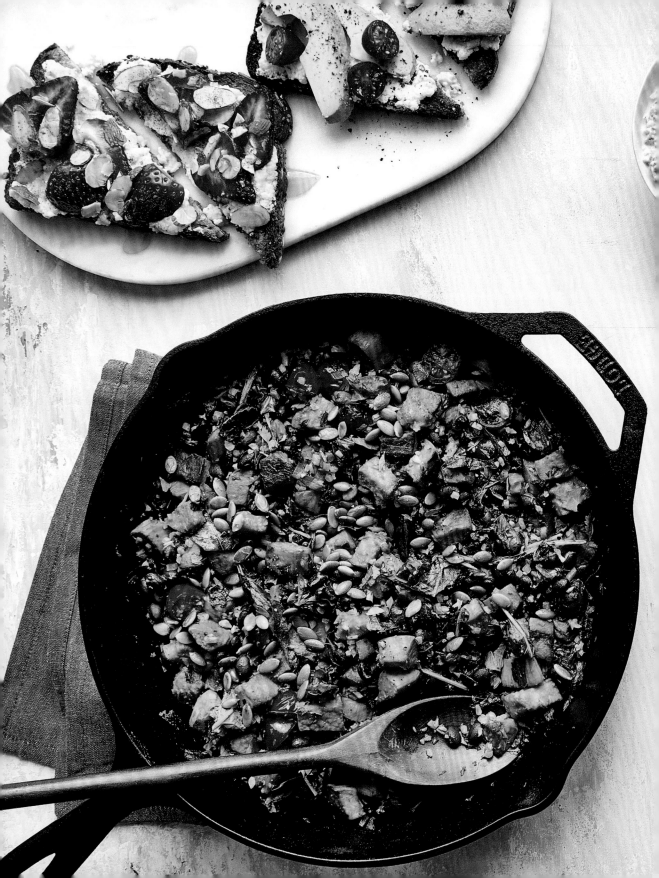

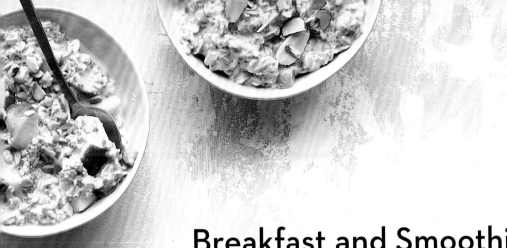

Breakfast and Smoothies

Green Apple Pie Protein Smoothie

One of my favorite things to make are smoothies because there are literally endless combinations you can try, they take minutes to make, and you can pack a ton of nutritious ingredients into them while keeping calories in check. Each ingredient in this delicious recipe provides weight-management and blood-pressure-lowering benefits. Rich in protein, potassium, calcium, magnesium, healthy fats, and fiber, this creamy meal in a glass will jump-start your day with a healthy dose of nutrition.

¾ cup unsweetened vanilla almond or cashew milk

2 tablespoons oat bran

¼ teaspoon apple pie spice or ground cinnamon

½ teaspoon vanilla extract

1 cup baby spinach or ⅓ cup frozen (see Tips)

½ cup nonfat (0%) plain Greek yogurt

1 tablespoon avocado

½ medium banana, sliced and frozen

½ cup green apple, unpeeled, chopped and frozen (see Tips)

¼ cup cooked or canned white beans (see Tips), rinsed and drained

½ cup ice, or to desired consistency

In a high-powered blender, combine the milk, oat bran, apple pie spice, vanilla, spinach, avocado, banana, apple, beans, and ice. Blend until smooth. Serve immediately.

TIPS: For the spinach and apples, you can use either fresh or frozen. Frozen ingredients make a thicker smoothie, while fresh ingredients tend to produce a thinner smoothie, so when making substitutions, you will need to adjust the amount of liquid/ice you use.

Beans in a smoothie? Beans are actually a fantastic smoothie ingredient, not only for their health benefits of protein, fiber, minerals, and B vitamins, but also because they blend up nice and creamy you won't even notice they are there. I like using frozen green peas, frozen shelled edamame, and white beans because of their neutral taste. If I make a smoothie with cocoa or cacao, black beans are my bean of choice.

PER SERVING: Calories: 319; Total fat: 5 g; Saturated fat: <1 g; Cholesterol: 5 mg; Sodium: 226 mg; Potassium: 1,074 mg; Total carbohydrates: 50 g; Fiber: 10 g; Sugars: 19 g; Protein: 21 g

Chocolate-Cherry Smoothie Bowl

Smoothie bowls are extra-thick smoothies made by using less liquid than a traditional smoothie and are meant to be eaten with a spoon. Due to their richer and creamier consistency that is almost ice cream–like, and because they are eaten with a spoon and not a straw, you can load them up with all kinds of fabulous toppings. Cocoa and cherries are nutritionally dense foods rich in antioxidant phytochemicals, blood-pressure-lowering minerals, and fiber for weight management. Hearty, wholesome, and delicious, this smoothie bowl is a quick and delicious way to start your day.

SMOOTHIE

½ cup unsweetened vanilla almond or cashew milk

1 teaspoon vanilla extract

1 cup fresh baby spinach or ⅓ cup frozen (see Tips)

1 tablespoon almond butter

1 tablespoon unsweetened cocoa powder

½ cup nonfat (0%) plain Greek yogurt

¾ cup frozen cherries

½ medium banana, sliced and frozen

3 to 4 ice cubes, or to desired consistency

FOR SERVING

½ small banana, sliced

¼ cup berries, such as blueberries, raspberries, or strawberries

1 teaspoon sliced almonds

½ tablespoon cacao nibs

1. Make the smoothie: In a high-powered blender, combine the milk, vanilla, spinach, almond butter, cocoa, yogurt, cherries, banana, and ice. Blend until thick and creamy.

2. To serve, pour into a bowl and top with the sliced banana, berries, sliced almonds, and cacao nibs. Enjoy immediately.

TIPS: For an even thicker smoothie, try adding some chia gel. Chia seeds are rich in heart-healthy omega-3 fats, antioxidants, fiber, and chia gel, which is a nutritious thickener. To make chia gel, an ideal ratio is ⅓ cup chia seeds to 2 cups water. Put the water into a container with a tight-fitting lid and pour the seeds into the water. Cover and shake for 15 seconds. Let stand for 1 minute, then shake again and refrigerate until it forms a gel, about 10 minutes. The gel will keep in the refrigerator for 2 weeks.

When substituting frozen for fresh spinach, keep in mind that the frozen spinach is much more concentrated, and if you use too much, it will overpower your dish. Use only one-third the amount of fresh called for: In this case, ⅓ cup frozen for 1 cup fresh.

PER SERVING: Calories: 412; Total fat: 14 g; Saturated fat: 2 g; Cholesterol: 5 mg; Sodium: 182 mg; Potassium: 1,416 mg; Total carbohydrates: 61 g; Fiber: 13 g; Sugars: 35 g; Protein: 20 g

Strawberry Orange Beet Smoothie

Beets are an amazing addition to your diet because they are packed full of nutrients and deliver a one-two punch of blood-pressure-lowering nutrients. Beets are rich in nitrates, which the body converts into nitric oxide, a compound that relaxes and dilates blood vessels, which means better circulation and lower blood pressure. They are also high in folate and phytochemicals, nutrients that keep levels of homocysteine, which increase your risk for heart disease, in check. Vibrant, sweet, and filling, this nutrient-rich smoothie is full of protein, vitamin C, calcium, and healthy omega-3 fats, making it a quick and easy breakfast for weight loss and heart health. Prepare your taste buds for a unique and distinctively delicious-tasting smoothie!

¾ cup unsweetened almond milk

1 tablespoon hemp seeds

1 teaspoon honey

½ teaspoon vanilla extract

½ cup nonfat (0%) plain Greek yogurt (see Tips)

½ cup frozen strawberries

½ navel orange, peeled, quartered, and frozen

½ cup sliced cooked beets (if using canned, use no-salt-added beets)

3 to 4 ice cubes

In a high-powered blender, combine the almond milk and hemp seeds and blend on low for 20 to 30 seconds. Add the honey, vanilla, yogurt, strawberries, orange, beets, and ice. Blend until thick and creamy. Serve immediately.

TIPS: If you like your smoothies extra thick and creamy, add ¼ to ½ teaspoon of xanthan and/or guar gum. Gums are in all kinds of foods as binders. Guar gum is generally recommended for cold foods like ice cream, and xanthan gum for baked goods, but I find that when you use them together they have a synergistic effect and add both volume and a creamy consistency. You can find them in the baking aisle.

You can make any of the smoothie recipes vegan and retain the heart-health benefits by swapping out the Greek yogurt for an equal amount of calcium-fortified tofu or a plant-based yogurt, or even a plant-based protein powder like pea, rice, or hemp protein.

PER SERVING: Calories: 251; Total fat: 6 g; Saturated fat: <1 g; Cholesterol: 5 mg; Sodium: 239 mg; Potassium: 721 mg; Total carbohydrates: 32 g; Fiber: 7 g; Sugars: 18 g; Protein: 17 g

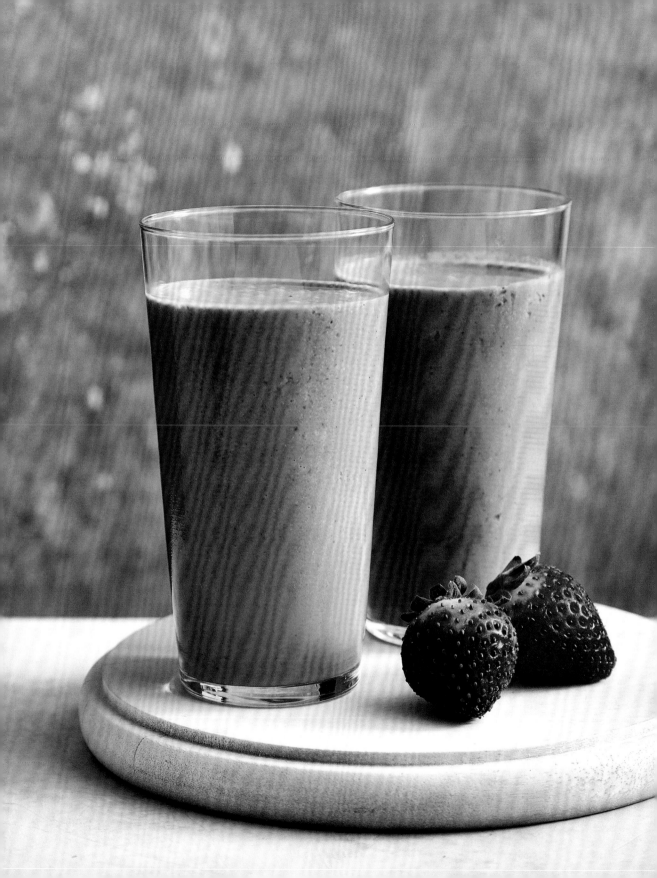

PREP TIME: 5 MINUTES • COOK TIME: 35 MINUTES • SERVES 4

Blueberry-Walnut Steel-Cut Oats

Steel-cut oats are a power food that should be a regular part of your diet. They provide long-lasting energy, weight-management benefits, and heart-healthy vitamins and minerals. An excellent source of protein and soluble and insoluble fiber, steel-cut oats provide a sustained release of energy to maintain satiety through the morning. With the addition of antioxidant- and phytochemical-rich blueberries and healthy fats from walnuts, this recipe is certain to become a family favorite.

1 cup fat-free dairy milk or almond milk or soy milk

1 cup steel-cut oats

Pinch of salt

½ teaspoon ground cinnamon

1 cup fresh blueberries, rinsed and drained (can substitute frozen)

¼ cup chopped walnuts

Sweetener of choice (optional)

1. In a large saucepan, combine the milk and 2 to 3 cups water (see Tip). Bring to a boil over medium heat. Stir in the steel-cut oats and salt.

2. Reduce the heat to medium-low and cook for 30 minutes, stirring occasionally to prevent sticking. Keep an eye on the pot as oats tend to boil over if the heat is too high. When the oats start to thicken, stir in the cinnamon and blueberries.

3. Portion into 4 bowls and serve the oats hot topped with chopped walnuts. Add a sweetener, if desired.

TIP: The basic ratio for making steel-cut oatmeal is 1 cup oats to 3 to 4 cups liquid. If you like your oats more intact and chewier, use only 3 cups. If you like a silkier porridge, use 4 cups. Experiment to find the consistency you enjoy the most. Leftover oats will keep in the refrigerator for up to 1 week, so you can make a big pot on the weekend and have breakfast prepped for the week.

PER SERVING: Calories: 241; Total fat: 7 g; Saturated fat: 1 g; Cholesterol: 1 mg; Sodium: 48 mg; Potassium: 164 mg; Total carbohydrates: 37 g; Fiber: 6 g; Sugars: 8 g; Protein: 8 g

Overnight Oats Three Ways

Overnight oats keep well in the refrigerator for up to 5 days, so you can prep a week's worth of breakfasts on a Sunday and enjoy a healthy, nutritious, fuss-free breakfast all week long. Packed with satiating whole-grain goodness and fiber, here are three variations packed with delicious blood-pressure-lowering foods.

Apple-Pistachio Overnight Oats

- ½ cup rolled oats
- 1 tablespoon chia seeds
- ½ cup fat-free milk
- ¼ cup nonfat (0%) plain Greek yogurt
- ¼ teaspoon vanilla extract
- ¼ teaspoon ground cinnamon
- 1 teaspoon honey or maple syrup
- ½ cup apple, washed, unpeeled, chopped
- 1 tablespoon unsalted pistachios, for serving

Pumpkin-Flax Overnight Oats

- ½ cup rolled oats
- 1 tablespoon flaxseed meal
- ½ cup fat-free milk
- ¼ cup nonfat (0%) plain Greek yogurt
- ¼ teaspoon vanilla extract
- ¼ teaspoon pumpkin pie spice
- 1 teaspoon honey or maple syrup
- ¼ cup canned unsweetened pumpkin puree
- 1 tablespoon pumpkin seeds, for serving

Raspberry Mango Turmeric Overnight Oats

- ½ cup rolled oats
- 1 tablespoon chia seeds
- ½ cup fat-free milk
- ¼ cup nonfat (0%) plain Greek yogurt
- ¼ teaspoon vanilla extract
- ¼ teaspoon ground turmeric
- ¼ teaspoon ground ginger
- 1 teaspoon honey or maple syrup
- ½ cup frozen raspberries
- ¼ cup frozen mango cut into chunks
- 2 teaspoons sliced almonds, for serving

1. In a jar or bowl, combine the oats, chia seeds or flaxseed meal, milk, yogurt, vanilla, spices, sweetener, and fruit and stir to combine.

2. Cover and place in the refrigerator for at least 4 hours or overnight.

3. When you are ready to serve, remove from the refrigerator, stir, and add additional milk if the oats are too thick.

4. Top with nuts/seeds and serve chilled or warm in the microwave.

Continued

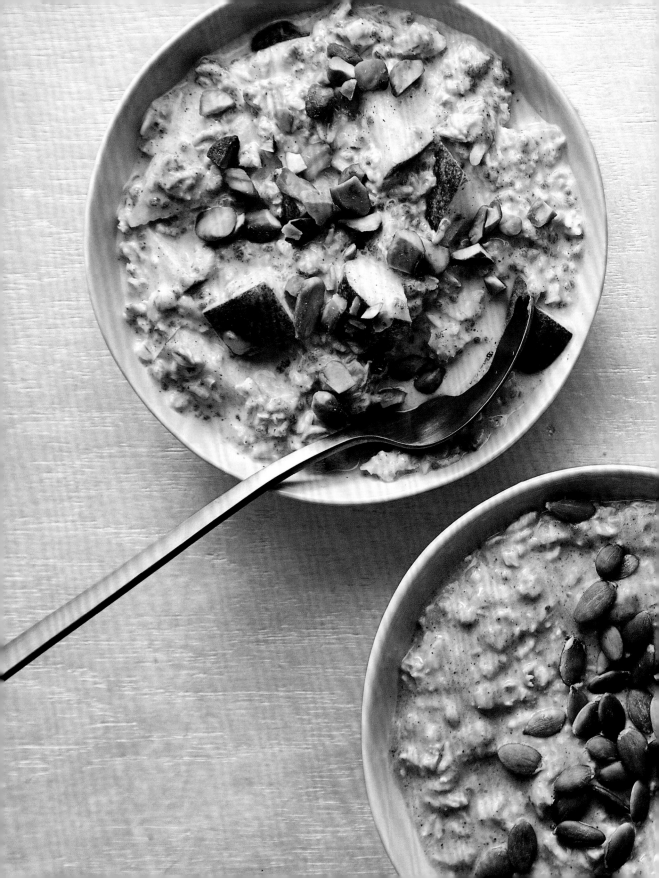

APPLE-PISTACHIO
PER SERVING: Calories: 410; Total fat: 10 g; Saturated fat: <1 g; Cholesterol: 5 mg; Sodium: 81 mg; Potassium: 451 mg; Total carbohydrates: 57 g; Fiber: 10 g; Sugars: 22 g; Protein: 20 g

PUMPKIN-FLAX
PER SERVING: Calories: 345; Total fat: 10 g; Saturated fat: 1 g; Cholesterol: 5 mg; Sodium: 84 mg; Potassium: 324 mg; Total carbohydrates: 49 g; Fiber: 9 g; Sugars: 18 g; Protein: 20 g

RASPBERRY MANGO TURMERIC
PER SERVING: Calories: 405; Total fat: 10 g; Saturated fat: <1 g; Cholesterol: 5 mg; Sodium: 82 mg; Potassium: 565 mg; Total carbohydrates: 64 g; Fiber: 15 g; Sugars: 24 g; Protein: 20 g

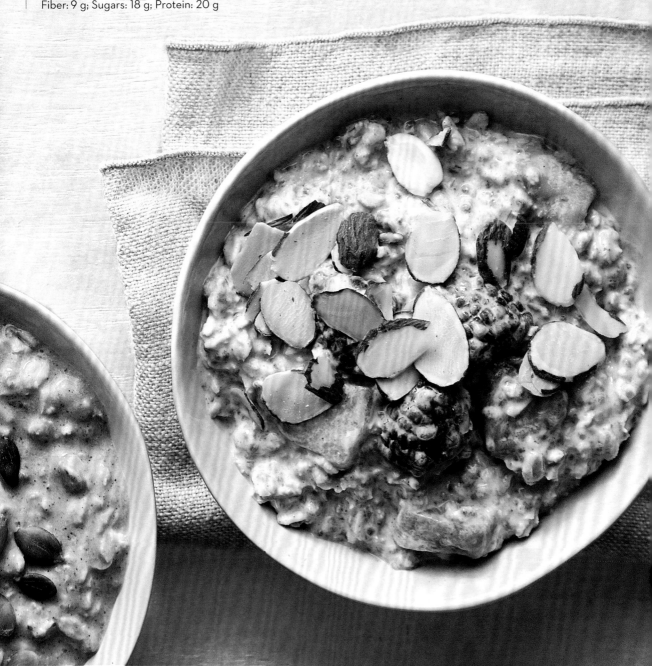

Apricot-Banana Breakfast Barley

Barley is one of those highly underrated grains—it is lower in calories and higher in fiber and protein than most other grains. Barley is rich in a particular type of fiber called beta-glucan, which lowers bad cholesterol, and is an excellent source of calcium, potassium, magnesium, and B vitamins. Bananas are packed with potassium and prebiotics that help balance the bacteria in your gut, apricots add vitamin C, potassium, fiber, and phytochemicals, while almonds add a dose of healthy fats. Creamy, filling, and delicious, breakfast barley can help you achieve your weight-loss and heart-health goals.

1 cup pearl barley, rinsed and drained (see Tip)

1 to 1½ cups fat-free milk or plant-based milk

Pinch of salt

4 dried apricots, finely chopped

1 large banana, sliced

4 teaspoons sliced almonds

Sweetener of choice (optional)

1. In a 4-quart saucepan, combine the barley, 2 cups water, 1 cup of the milk, the salt, apricots, and banana. Bring to a boil over high heat, then reduce the heat to low. Cover and cook until most of the liquid is absorbed, about 30 minutes. Add an additional ½ cup milk, if necessary, to reach desired consistency.

2. Portion into 4 bowls and top with sliced almonds and a sweetener, if desired.

TIP: "Hull-less" or hulled barley is the least processed and most nutritious form of this grain, but it can be hard to find and you may need to order it online. While pearl barley is a bit less nutritious because it has had most of the outer grain removed, it is readily available in grocery stores, cooks quickly, and still boasts a great deal of fiber.

PER SERVING (WITHOUT THE EXTRA ½ CUP MILK): Calories: 258; Total fat: 2 g; Saturated fat: <1 g; Cholesterol: 1 mg; Sodium: 51 mg; Potassium: 457 mg; Total carbohydrates: 55 g; Fiber: 9 g; Sugars: 11 g; Protein: 8 g

Creamy Peach Quinoa

Quinoa is a super-nutritious whole grain that has gone mainstream in the last couple of years and is readily available in grocery stores. One of the few plant sources of complete protein, quinoa has all of the essential amino acids your body needs, plus it is a good source of fiber and an excellent source of magnesium and manganese. The best part is that quinoa cooks up quickly, and the tiny round grains pop and expand to produce a chewy satisfying texture. This recipe uses fresh peaches for added nutrients and fiber, and walnuts for healthy fats, but feel free to use your favorite fruit and nuts.

1 cup quinoa, rinsed and drained (see Tip)

2 cups fat-free milk

1 cup finely chopped peaches

1/2 teaspoon ground cinnamon

Pinch of salt

2 tablespoons chopped walnuts

Sweetener of choice (optional)

TIP: Most recipes suggest you rinse quinoa before using to remove the bitter coating on the outside of the seeds, called saponin, which can make it taste bitter. However, most commercially available quinoa is prerinsed.

1. In a medium saucepan, combine the quinoa, milk, peaches, cinnamon, and salt. Stir to combine, bring to a boil, covered. Reduce the heat to medium-low and cook, covered, until most of the liquid has been absorbed, about 20 minutes.

2. Remove the saucepan from the heat and let stand, covered, 5 minutes. Fluff with a fork.

3. Portion into 4 bowls and top each with 1/2 tablespoon chopped walnuts and sweetener, if desired.

PER SERVING: Calories: 245; Total fat: 5 g; Saturated fat: <1 g; Cholesterol: 2 mg; Sodium: 81 mg; Potassium: 293 mg; Total carbohydrates: 41 g; Fiber: 4 g; Sugars: 10 g; Protein: 11 g

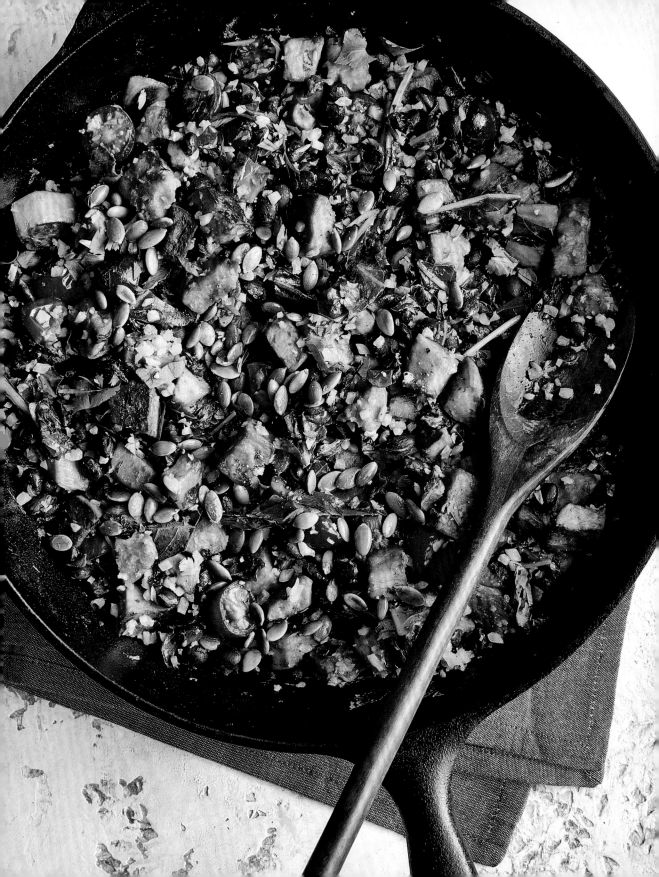

Quick Skillet Sweet Potato and Black Bean Hash

Our health would benefit by taking cues from the many cultures around the world where beans are a staple on the breakfast menu. Beans are packed with plant protein, blood sugar–stabilizing and appetite-squashing fiber, B vitamins, and minerals. Sweet potatoes are an equally nutritious food and are rich in beta-carotene, which raises blood levels of vitamin A, and vitamin C, B vitamins, potassium, fiber, and antioxidants. Cooked together in one skillet with vegetables and spices, this hearty and satisfying dish is simple to make and is packed with flavor.

1 tablespoon extra-virgin olive oil

1 cup diced peeled sweet potato (see Tips)

1 (15-ounce) can black beans, rinsed and drained

1 cup riced cauliflower

4 cherry tomatoes, halved

2 cups baby kale, stems removed, finely chopped, or substitute ⅔ cup frozen (see Tips)

1 teaspoon sweet paprika

Pinch of freshly ground black pepper

1 ounce (about 3 tablespoons) unsalted roasted pumpkin seeds

¼ cup chopped fresh cilantro

1. In a medium saucepan, heat the oil over medium-high heat until shimmering, about 30 seconds. Add the sweet potato and cook, stirring frequently until softened and lightly browned, about 5 minutes.

2. Stir in the beans, riced cauliflower, tomatoes, kale, paprika, and black pepper and continue cooking over medium heat until the beans are heated and the kale has wilted, about 5 minutes.

3. Remove from the heat and portion onto 3 plates. Top with the pumpkin seeds and cilantro.

PER SERVING: Calories: 298; Total fat: 10 g; Saturated fat: 2 g; Cholesterol: 0 mg; Sodium: 45 mg; Potassium: 521 mg; Total carbohydrates: 42 g; Fiber: 12 g; Sugars: 5 g; Protein: 14 g

TIPS: You can find prewashed and cubed sweet potato and riced cauliflower in the produce aisle, which can cut down on prep time. Feel free to mix up the vegetables based on what you have on hand.

When substituting frozen greens for fresh, use a ratio of roughly 1:3 (frozen to fresh). The frozen greens are much more concentrated, so you only need to use one-third the volume. If you use too much, it will overpower the dish.

Ricotta Breakfast Toast Two Ways

An essential part of any weight-management plan is consistency in when and how you fuel your body. By taking just 10 minutes each morning to prepare a quick and nutritious breakfast, you will have the energy to conquer your day, keep cravings at bay, and be more successful as you work toward your weight-loss goals. Creamy ricotta cheese is an excellent source of protein and calcium, and when coupled with a serving of whole-grain bread, fruits, veggies, and healthy fats, creates a perfect light breakfast.

Strawberry Almond Ricotta Toast

1 slice hearty whole-grain bread (Dave's Killer 21 Whole Grains and Seeds or any 100% whole-grain bread)

1/3 cup part-skim ricotta cheese

1 teaspoon honey

1/2 cup sliced strawberries

1 tablespoon sliced almonds

Pinch of ground cinnamon

1. Toast the bread to your liking.

2. Spread with the ricotta cheese, drizzle with the honey, layer the strawberries on top, and sprinkle with the almonds and cinnamon.

PER SERVING: Calories: 286; Total fat: 10 g; Saturated fat: 3 g; Cholesterol: 26 mg; Sodium: 379 mg; Potassium: 300 mg; Total carbohydrates: 38 g; Fiber: 8 g; Sugars: 17 g; Protein: 16 g

TIP: Take this recipe and put your own DASH healthy spin on it. For example, try 2 tablespoons of hummus with cucumber slices or apple slices; 2 tablespoons of low-fat (2%) Greek yogurt and 1 tablespoon of pumpkin seeds; or 2 tablespoons mashed white beans, black pepper, and 1 tablespoon chopped walnuts. Having a repertoire of quick and easy recipes that you can customize means you never get bored and can create sweet or savory toast depending on your mood.

Avocado Tomato Ricotta Toast

1 slice hearty whole-grain bread (Dave's Killer 21 Whole Grains and Seeds or any 100% whole-grain bread)

1/3 cup part-skim ricotta cheese

1/2 cup avocado, sliced

4 cherry tomatoes, halved

1/2 lemon

Pinch of freshly ground black pepper

1. Toast the bread to your liking.

2. Spread the bread with the ricotta cheese, layer the avocado slices on top, arrange the tomato halves on top of the avocado, then top with a squeeze of lemon and a dash of black pepper.

PER SERVING: Calories: 366; Total fat: 20 g; Saturated fat: 4 g; Cholesterol: 26 mg; Sodium: 384 mg; Potassium: 686 mg; Total carbohydrates: 39 g; Fiber: 9 g; Sugars: 7 g; Protein: 18 g

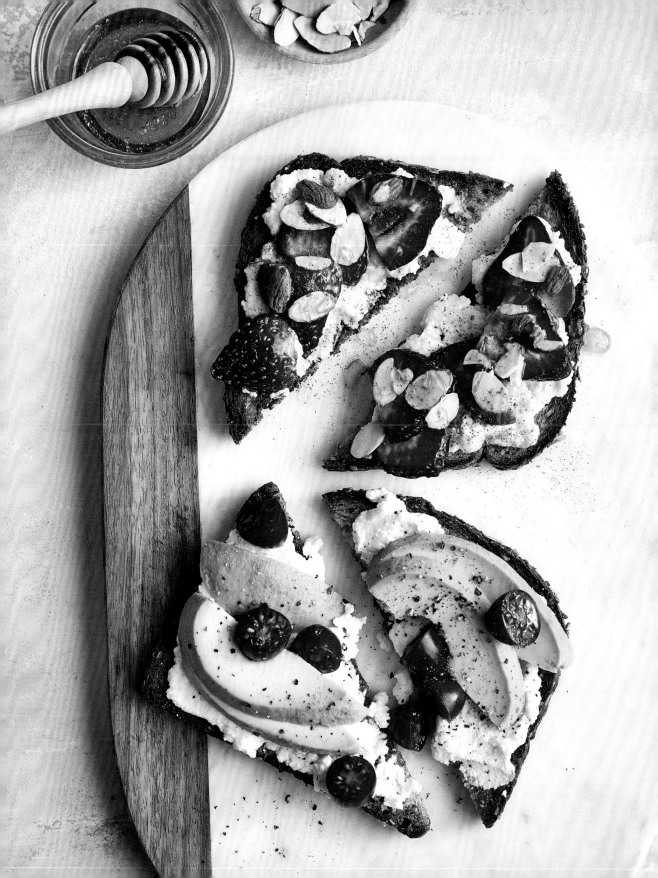

2-Minute Egg and Vegetable Breakfast Mug

This quick and easy microwave egg-and-vegetable mug recipe is perfect for busy mornings, and is customizable based on the ingredients you have on hand or dietary preferences. Just as fluffy as an omelet made on the stovetop, simply pair this with a bowl of berries for added fiber and a nutrient-rich, energizing breakfast.

2 eggs (see Tips)

2 tablespoons fat-free milk or plant-based milk

¼ cup thinly sliced spinach

2 cherry tomatoes, halved

2 tablespoons chopped mushroom

4 frozen broccoli florets, chopped

½ teaspoon dried basil

Freshly ground black pepper

Optional toppings: salsa, sliced avocado, shredded cheese

TIPS: Mugs that are wider and shorter work best. Be careful not to overcook, because the eggs will continue to cook and firm up after they are removed from the microwave.

The yolk contains most of the nutrients in an egg, including protein, the fat-soluble vitamins A, D, E, and K, essential fatty acids, carotenoids, B vitamins, and choline. However, you can make this recipe lower in calories by using 1 whole egg and 2 egg whites.

1. Spray the inside of a large microwave-safe mug (see Tips), custard cup, or ramekin with cooking spray.

2. Add the eggs and milk to the mug and using a fork, mix until the yolks are combined. Fill the mug two-thirds full (don't fill to the brim), because the eggs will fluff up and expand during the cooking process.

3. Add the spinach, tomatoes, mushroom, broccoli, basil, and pepper to taste. Gently stir to combine.

4. Transfer the mug to the microwave and cook on high for 1 minute.

5. Stir the mixture and microwave for an additional minute or until the eggs are almost set. Cooking times will vary depending on your microwave's strength.

6. Sprinkle with optional toppings, if desired.

PER SERVING: Calories: 175; Total fat: 10 g; Saturated fat: 3 g; Cholesterol: 373 mg; Sodium: 169 mg; Potassium: 386 mg; Total carbohydrates: 6 g; Fiber: 1 g; Sugars: 3 g; Protein: 15 g

Banana-Almond Pancakes for One

Pancakes shouldn't be complicated, and they definitely don't have to be heavy and loaded in calories. This recipe requires only a handful of nutritious ingredients, and simplifies things by eliminating the mixing bowl and whisk. Simply throw your ingredients into a blender and cook them on the stovetop in minutes. While not fluffy like traditional pancakes, they have a hearty, satisfying texture and are super nutritious, with ample amounts of potassium, fiber, and protein. Although this recipe is written for one, you can easily double or triple the recipe to fit your household.

1 medium banana, sliced

2 large eggs

2 tablespoons almond meal/flour (see Tip)

2 tablespoons quick oats

1 teaspoon almond butter (see Tip)

½ teaspoon baking powder

¼ cup raspberries, washed and drained

TIP: You can customize this recipe by changing up the type of flour and nut butter, using what you have on hand. Try peanut butter and ½ cup oat bran in place of the flours, or use ½ cup buckwheat flour with walnut butter for an earthier, heartier texture and taste.

1. In a high-powered blender, combine the banana, eggs, almond meal/flour, oats, almond butter, and baking powder and process until smooth. (Don't worry if the batter seems too thin; the pancakes will cook up perfectly.)

2. Coat a skillet with cooking spray and set over medium heat.

3. Pour the batter in 2-tablespoon amounts onto the pan and let cook for about 1 minute. Flip and cook on the other side until lightly browned and firm, about 1 minute more.

4. Serve topped with fresh berries.

PER SERVING: Calories: 414; Total fat: 21 g; Saturated fat: 4 g; Cholesterol: 372 mg; Sodium: 146 mg; Potassium: 898 mg; Total carbohydrates: 43 g; Fiber: 8 g; Sugars: 17 g; Protein: 19 g

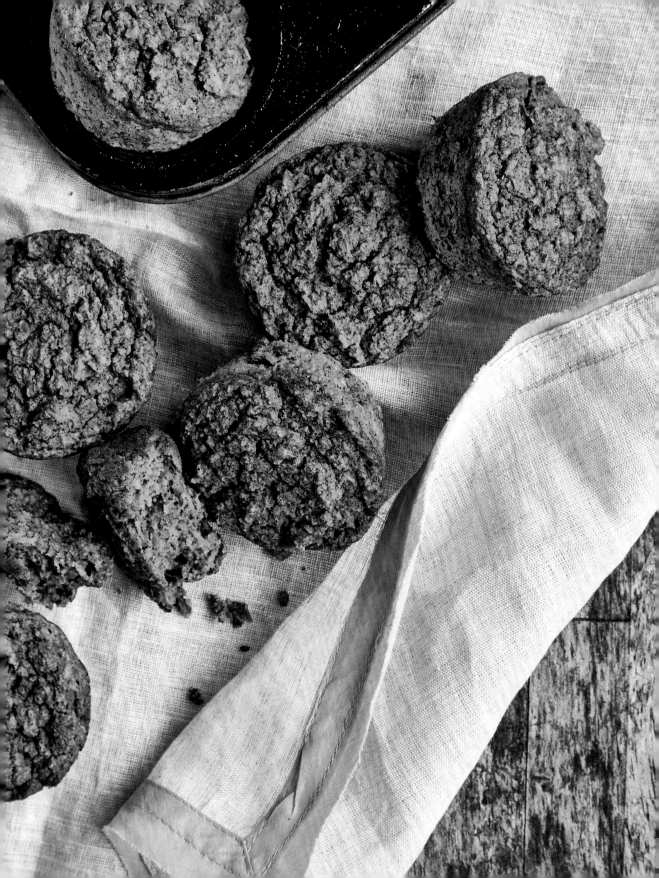

High-Protein Apple Carrot Hemp Muffins

I developed this recipe for my mom a number of years ago when she was trying to get her cholesterol in check. She also has a tendency to skip breakfast, so I wanted her to have a recipe that she could make and have on hand for breakfasts and snacks throughout the week. Apples are high in pectin (which has cholesterol-lowering benefits), the Greek yogurt adds protein and calcium, the hemp adds healthy omega-3 fatty acids and fiber, and the carrots boost the fiber, vitamin, and mineral content. These moist muffins are super delicious, freeze well, and are quick to prepare.

1 cup nonfat (0%) plain Greek yogurt

2 cups shredded carrots

4 cups diced unpeeled apples

1½ cups oat flour

½ cup plain high-fiber hemp protein (see Tip)

½ cup granulated no-calorie sweetener

1 tablespoon ground nutmeg

1 teaspoon baking soda

1 teaspoon baking powder

¼ teaspoon salt

½ cup liquid egg whites

TIP: Plant-based protein powders are an easy and nutritious way to boost the protein content of a meal, and, depending on the source, the fiber content. Hemp protein works really well in baking and can be substituted for up to one-quarter of the flour in recipes. Hemp protein is easy to find in grocery stores, big box retailers, and online. Pea protein can be substituted and will produce similar results.

1. Preheat the oven to 350°F. Coat 12 cups of a standard muffin tin with cooking spray.

2. In a blender, combine the yogurt, carrots, and apples and blend until it has the consistency of applesauce.

3. In a medium bowl, combine the oat flour, hemp protein, no-calorie sweetener, nutmeg, baking soda, baking powder, and salt and stir to combine.

4. Add the egg whites to the dry ingredients followed by the pureed yogurt/carrot/apple mixture and mix thoroughly.

5. Portion the batter evenly into the muffin cups, filling each about two-thirds full with batter.

6. Bake until a toothpick inserted into the center comes out clean, about 20 minutes. Remove from the oven and allow the muffins to cool on a wire rack. They freeze really well for up to 2 months and will keep in the refrigerator for up to one week.

PER MUFFIN: Calories: 123; Total fat: 2 g; Saturated fat: <1 g; Cholesterol: <1 mg; Sodium: 193 mg; Potassium: 340 mg; Total carbohydrates: 21 g; Fiber: 5 g; Sugars: 6 g; Protein: 9 g

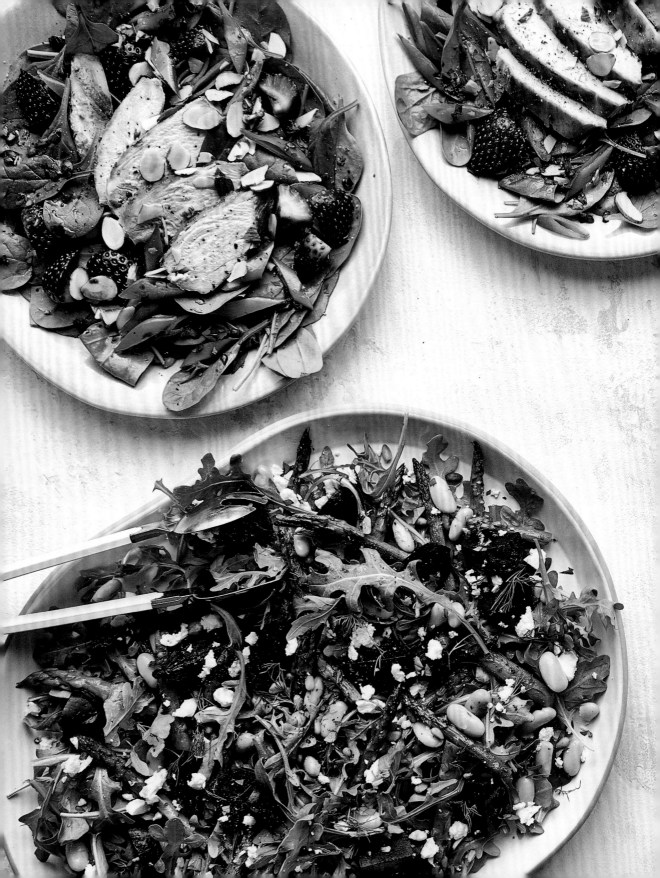

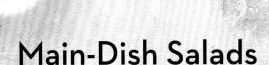

Main-Dish Salads

Roasted Salmon, Spinach, and Butternut Squash Salad

Salmon is one of the most nutritious foods you can include in your heart-healthy diet. It's rich in nutrients that can lower your risk for heart disease, and can help you to manage your weight. This fatty fish is an excellent source of the essential long-chain omega-3 fatty acids EPA and DHA, which have been shown to reduce inflammation, lower blood pressure, and reduce the risk for certain cancers. Salmon is also rich in potassium as well as numerous other minerals, B vitamins, and antioxidants. This simple recipe bakes salmon with creamy, potassium- and fiber-rich butternut squash, and dresses the fish and vegetables with a delicious and light tarragon dressing.

1 (16-ounce) package diced peeled butternut squash (see Tip)

4 tablespoons extra-virgin olive oil

Salt and freshly ground black pepper

4 skinless salmon fillets (6 ounces each)

3 tablespoons fresh lemon juice

2 cloves garlic, minced

1 tablespoon minced fresh tarragon or 1 teaspoon dried

1 teaspoon Dijon mustard

8 cups baby spinach

TIP: You can find peeled and precut butternut squash in the produce section of the grocery store. Buying the precut squash is both economical and efficient—if you have ever prepped your own diced squash from a whole unpeeled squash, you know it requires a certain amount of muscle and time.

1. Preheat the oven to 425°F. Line a rimmed baking sheet with foil.

2. In a medium bowl, toss the squash with 1 tablespoon of the olive oil, a pinch of salt, and ¼ teaspoon pepper. Spread on the prepared baking sheet and roast, stirring once, for 15 minutes.

3. Remove the pan from the oven (leave the oven on) and move the squash to one side. Place the salmon fillets on the foil and sprinkle each with salt and pepper, if desired. Return to the oven and bake until the salmon flakes easily with a fork, 5 to 10 minutes, turning halfway through the cooking time.

4. Meanwhile, in a small bowl, whisk together the lemon juice, remaining 3 tablespoons olive oil, the garlic, tarragon, and Dijon mustard.

5. In a large bowl, add the spinach and half of the vinaigrette and toss to combine. Portion the spinach onto 4 serving plates, top with one-quarter of the butternut squash and salmon fillet. Drizzle with some of the vinaigrette.

PER SERVING: Calories: 398; Total fat: 21 g; Saturated fat: 3 g; Cholesterol: 127 mg; Sodium: 185 mg; Potassium: 699 mg; Total carbohydrates: 16 g; Fiber: 5 g; Sugars: 3 g; Protein: 37 g

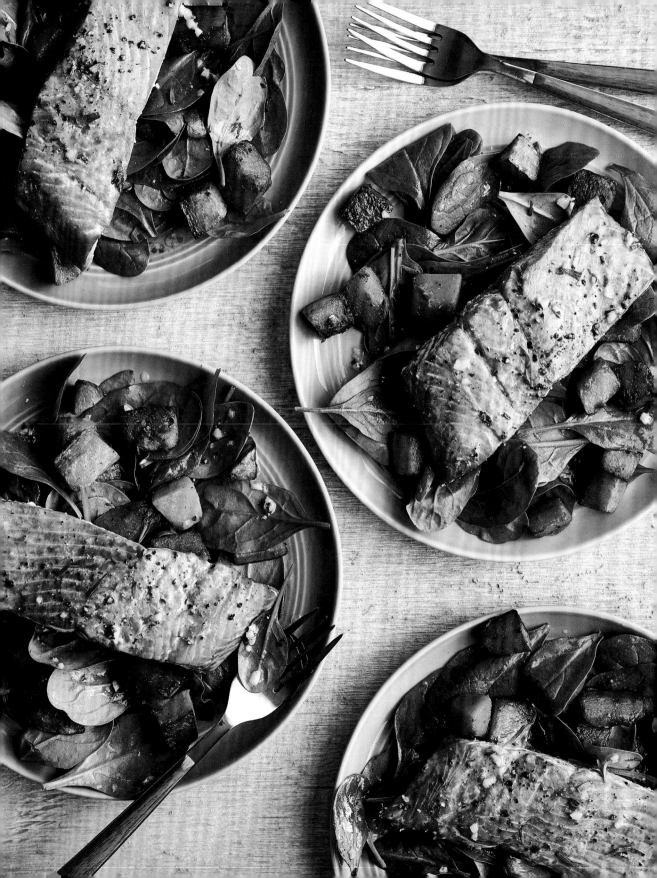

Barley and Roasted Brussels Sprouts with Fresh Herbs and Ricotta

Fiber-rich barley is mixed with roasted Brussels sprouts and cranberry beans in this filling and protein-rich recipe. Fresh herbs and a lemony vinaigrette add bright flavors, and the dish is finished with a garnish of creamy, calcium-rich ricotta. Wholesome and delicious, this nutritious recipe is a balanced meal perfect for those busy weeknights.

BARLEY

1 cup pearl barley

Pinch of salt

2 large cloves garlic, peeled but whole

BRUSSELS SPROUTS AND BEANS

1 pound Brussels sprouts, ends trimmed, halved

1 tablespoon + 1 teaspoon extra-virgin olive oil

Freshly ground black pepper (optional)

1 (15-ounce) can cranberry or small red beans, rinsed and drained

1/4 cup finely sliced fresh chives

Pinch of salt

VINAIGRETTE

1 teaspoon finely grated lemon zest

1 tablespoon fresh lemon juice

2 shallots (see Tip), finely chopped (about 1/4 cup)

Freshly ground black pepper (optional)

2 tablespoons balsamic vinegar

3 tablespoons extra-virgin olive oil

FOR SERVING

1 cup part-skim ricotta cheese

1/4 cup chopped fresh parsley

Extra-virgin olive oil, for drizzling (optional)

Freshly ground black pepper

1. Make the barley: In a medium pot, bring 6 cups water to a boil over high heat. Add the barley, salt, and garlic. Reduce the heat to medium and simmer uncovered until firm-tender, 30 to 35 minutes. Drain well, discard the garlic, and let cool for 10 minutes.

2. Meanwhile, prepare the Brussels sprouts and beans: Preheat the oven to 400°F. Line a rimmed baking sheet with foil.

3. In a medium bowl, toss the Brussels sprouts with 1 tablespoon of the oil to coat. Sprinkle with pepper, if desired, and toss again. Spread out on the lined baking sheet and roast until the leaves are dark brown and crisp and the cut sides of the sprouts are browned, 20 to 25 minutes.

4. While the Brussels sprouts roast, place the beans in a microwave-safe dish with 1/4 cup water and heat for 1 minute or until warm. Drain and transfer to a large bowl.

5. Add the Brussels sprouts, chives, salt, and remaining 1 teaspoon olive oil to the beans.

6. Make the vinaigrette: In a small bowl, whisk together the lemon zest, lemon juice, shallots, pepper, if desired, vinegar, and oil until well blended.

7. Add the warm barley to the beans and Brussels sprouts. Drizzle with the vinaigrette and mix well.

8. To serve, divide among 4 serving bowls and top each with ¼ cup ricotta cheese and some chopped parsley. Drizzle with olive oil, if desired, and freshly ground black pepper to taste.

TIP: Shallots are a variety of onion and bear a close resemblance to garlic in structure. Low in calories, shallots are rich in a type of antioxidant that may protect the body against developing certain cancers, heart disease, and diabetes. Full of flavor and low in calories, 1 tablespoon chopped shallots is high in blood-pressure-lowering potassium. If you have trouble finding shallots, substitute an equal amount of chopped onion or garlic depending on your preference.

PER SERVING: Calories: 532; Total fat: 19 g; Saturated fat: 4 g; Cholesterol: 15 mg; Sodium: 131 mg; Potassium: 929 mg; Total carbohydrates: 74 g; Fiber: 19 g; Sugars: 8 g; Protein: 19 g

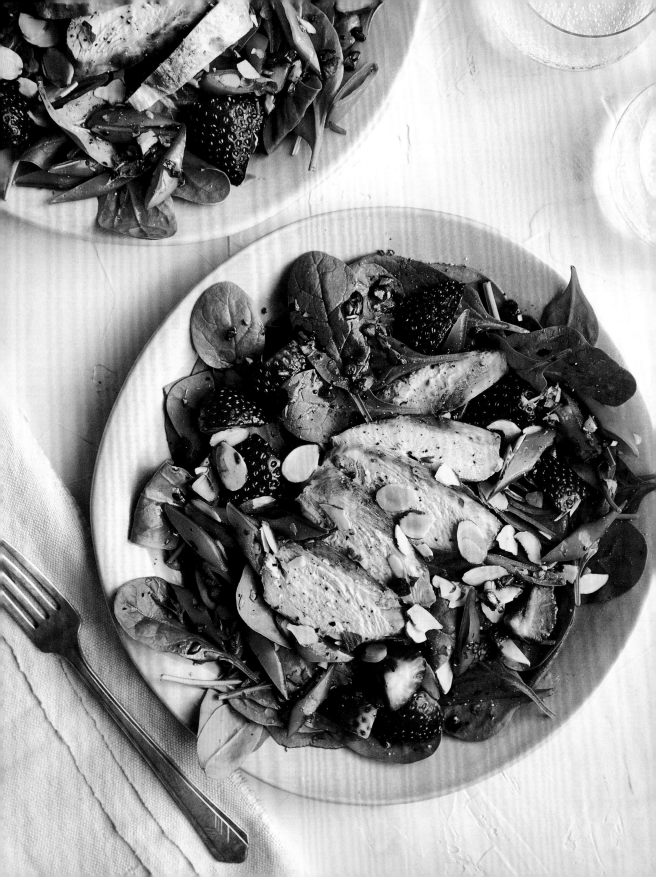

Strawberry Almond Chicken Salad with Crispy Snap Peas

Nutrient-rich salads are an excellent choice for any healthy eating plan. Simply use a base of fiber-rich greens, add 1 to 2 cups vegetables and a portion of protein, and dress your salad with a portion of healthy fats. This simple yet filling recipe dresses lean, protein-rich chicken breast with crispy snap peas, fresh strawberries, almonds, and fresh herbs.

CHICKEN

2 boneless, skinless chicken breasts (4 ounces each)

1 clove garlic, smashed with the side of knife

Pinch of salt

½ tablespoon extra-virgin olive oil

DRESSING

1 tablespoon extra-virgin olive oil

1 tablespoon balsamic vinegar

1 teaspoon honey

1 tablespoon finely chopped shallot

Freshly ground black pepper (optional)

¼ cup chopped fresh cilantro

SALAD

Pinch of salt

1 cup sugar snap peas, stems trimmed and cut on the diagonal into ¼-inch pieces

6 cups loosely packed baby spinach

1 cup strawberries, sliced

¼ cup sliced almonds

1. Prepare the chicken: Season the chicken with the smashed garlic and salt.

2. Heat a large skillet over medium heat and add the oil. When shimmering, add the chicken and cook until it lifts easily with a spatula, 4 to 5 minutes. Flip and continue cooking until a thermometer inserted in the center reads 165°F, another 4 to 5 minutes. Remove from the pan and set aside until cool, then slice.

3. Meanwhile, make the dressing: In a small bowl, whisk together the oil, vinegar, honey, 1 teaspoon water, the shallot, black pepper, if desired, and the cilantro. (See Tip.)

4. Make the salad: Bring a medium pot of water to a boil. Add the salt and the sugar snap peas and blanch until the peas are tender but still a bit crunchy, about 3 minutes. Drain and run under cold water and drain again. Pat dry to remove excess water.

5. In a large bowl, toss together the snap peas, spinach, strawberries, and almonds. Drizzle with the dressing and toss to combine.

6. Divide the salad between 2 serving plates. Slice the chicken and divide between the salads.

TIP: Store-bought salad dressings are extremely high in calories (100 to 200 calories per 2-tablespoon serving), salt, and unhealthy fats. It only takes a minute to prepare your own dressing by whisking together extra-virgin olive oil, vinegar, and fresh or dried herbs.

PER SERVING: Calories: 352; Total fat: 18 g; Saturated fat: 2 g; Cholesterol: 55 mg; Sodium: 307 mg; Potassium: 234 mg; Total carbohydrates: 20 g; Fiber: 6 g; Sugars: 9 g; Protein: 29 g

Simple Shrimp Salad for Two with Ginger Vinaigrette

Shrimp is an excellent source of vitamins and minerals including vitamin D, B vitamins, iron, zinc, and calcium. And while once thought to be bad for heart health due to their relatively high cholesterol content, researchers now know that it is saturated fat not dietary cholesterol that increases heart disease risk. Very low in calories and super quick to cook, this salad for two takes on an Asian flare with the addition of fiber and nutrient-rich green peas, colorful vegetables, and crunchy cashews, and is dressed in a healthy spicy ginger vinaigrette.

SALAD

1 cup frozen green peas

8 ounces peeled and deveined cooked shrimp, cut into ½-inch pieces

1 cup shredded carrots

1 medium red bell pepper, thinly sliced

¼ cup chopped cashews

2 tablespoons chopped scallions

GINGER DRESSING

2 tablespoons unseasoned rice vinegar

1 tablespoon extra-virgin olive oil (see Tip)

½ tablespoon sesame oil

2 tablespoons grated fresh ginger

1 teaspoon reduced-sodium soy sauce

Pinch of red pepper flakes

FOR SERVING

6 cups mixed baby greens

1. Prepare the salad: Bring a small pot of water to a boil. Add the peas and blanch until tender but not mushy, about 3 minutes. Drain and rinse under cold water until cool. Drain on paper towels, then transfer to a medium bowl.

2. To the bowl, add the shrimp, carrots, bell pepper, cashews, and scallions.

3. Make the ginger dressing: In a small bowl, whisk together the vinegar, extra-virgin olive oil, sesame oil, ginger, soy sauce, and pepper flakes.

4. Pour the dressing over the shrimp and vegetables and toss to coat.

5. To serve, divide the baby greens between 2 serving plates. Top with half of the shrimp/vegetable mixture.

TIP: Extra-virgin olive oil (EVOO) is typically more expensive than regular olive oil, but if you can afford it, it's the more nutritious of the two. EVOO is made by grinding olives into a paste and then pressing them to extract the oil with no heat involved. Regular olive oil is a blend including both processed and cold-pressed oils.

PER SERVING: Calories: 403; Total fat: 18 g; Saturated fat: 3 g; Cholesterol: 221 mg; Sodium: 568 mg; Potassium: 622 mg; Total carbohydrates: 23 g; Fiber: 9 g; Sugars: 7 g; Protein: 32 g

Quinoa and Spinach Power Salad

This vegan, gluten-free power salad is full of complete plant protein thanks to nutrient-rich quinoa, a seed containing all of the essential amino acids your body needs along with ample amounts of B vitamins, fiber, and minerals. A flavorful mix of nutritious ingredients with healthy fats and contrasting crunch (from almonds, snap peas, and cucumbers), chickpeas add plant protein and fiber, and spinach adds calcium, potassium, magnesium, and antioxidants to support a healthy heart. Topped with a simple, yet delicious, vinaigrette, this is a filling, colorful, and refreshing salad for two.

½ cup quinoa, rinsed and drained

2 cups spinach, finely chopped

1 medium tomato, diced

1 cup sugar snap peas

½ cup diced cucumbers

¼ cup sliced almonds

½ cup canned chickpeas, rinsed and drained

1½ tablespoons fresh lemon juice

1½ tablespoons extra-virgin olive oil

¼ teaspoon salt

¼ teaspoon freshly ground black pepper

TIP: Smaller amounts of quinoa such as used in this recipe take closer to 10 minutes to cook while larger amounts will be closer to 15 minutes.

1. In a medium saucepan, combine the quinoa and 1 cup water and bring to a boil over medium-high heat. Reduce the heat to a simmer, cover, and cook until the quinoa has absorbed all of the water, 10 to 15 minutes (see Tip).

2. Remove from the heat, cover, and let the quinoa steam for 5 minutes. Remove the lid and fluff with a fork.

3. In a large bowl, combine the spinach, tomato, snap peas, cucumbers, almonds, chickpeas, and cooled quinoa.

4. In a small bowl, whisk together the lemon juice, olive oil, salt, and pepper. Pour over the quinoa and vegetables and toss to coat.

5. Portion into 2 serving bowls.

PER SERVING: Calories: 439; Total fat: 20 g; Saturated fat: 2 g; Cholesterol: 0 mg; Sodium: 333 mg; Potassium: 565 mg; Total carbohydrates: 54 g; Fiber: 10 g; Sugars: 6 g; Protein: 15 g

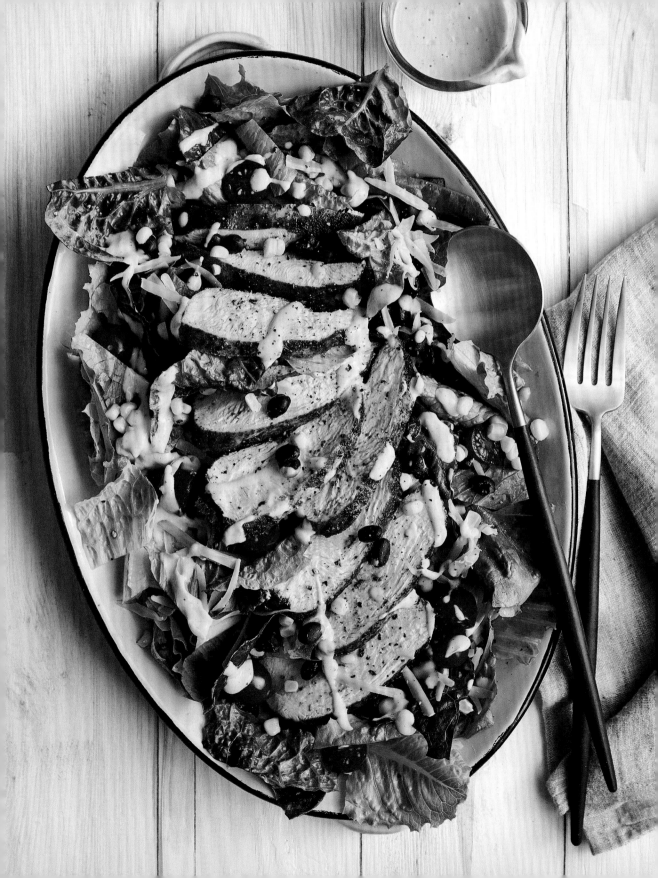

Southwestern Chicken Salad

This colorful protein- and fiber-rich salad comes together quickly to create a flavorful salad that will satisfy all of your Tex Mex cravings. Lean chicken breast is sautéed and sliced into strips and placed on top of a crunchy mix of vegetables and beans. Topped with a creamy avocado-cilantro dressing, this delicious meal is a perfect fit for your DASH weight-loss eating plan.

CHICKEN

2 boneless, skinless chicken breasts (4 ounces each)

1 teaspoon ground cumin

½ teaspoon chili powder

½ teaspoon paprika

Pinch of salt

1 tablespoon extra-virgin olive oil

SALAD

6 cups loosely packed chopped romaine lettuce

1 cup cherry tomatoes, halved

1 cup canned black beans, rinsed and drained

½ cup corn kernels

½ cup shredded low-fat cheddar cheese

DRESSING

½ avocado

2 tablespoons fresh lime juice

½ cup nonfat (0%) plain Greek yogurt

¼ cup packed fresh cilantro with stems (see Tips)

Pinch of salt

1. Cook the chicken: Season the chicken with cumin, chili powder, paprika, and salt.

2. Heat a large skillet over medium heat and add the olive oil. When shimmering, add the chicken to the pan and cook until it lifts easily with a spatula, 4 to 5 minutes. Flip and continue cooking until a thermometer inserted in the center reads 165°F, another 4 to 5 minutes. Remove from the pan and set aside.

3. Prepare the salad: In a large bowl, toss together the lettuce, tomatoes, beans, corn, and cheddar. Divide the salad among 4 serving plates.

4. Slice the chicken and divide among the salads.

5. Make the dressing: In a blender or food processor, combine the avocado, lime juice, Greek yogurt, cilantro, and salt and pulse for a few seconds until the cilantro is fully chopped. Top each salad plate with dressing.

TIPS: With its slightly tart taste, Greek yogurt makes a healthy, lower-calorie, higher-protein substitute for sour cream, mayonnaise, olive oil, and even heavy cream.

Cilantro is one of those strongly flavored herbs that people either love or hate. If you fall into the latter camp, feel free to substitute fresh parsley in its place.

PER SERVING: Calories: 273; Total fat: 11 g; Saturated fat: 3 g; Cholesterol: 39 mg; Sodium: 263 mg; Potassium: 572 mg; Total carbohydrates: 21 g; Fiber: 7 g; Sugars: 5 g; Protein: 24 g

Zucchini Noodle Mock Pasta Salad

Spiralized vegetables are pure genius in my opinion. They make eating healthier and keeping calories in check ridiculously easy. Zucchini noodles are versatile and can transform calorie-laden, refined carbohydrate-rich recipes into lightened-up, fiber-rich, and nutritious dishes. This zucchini noodle mock pasta salad is the perfect addition to a summer barbecue or potluck with its light and fresh taste. Packed with plant-powered protein from two types of beans and dressed in a creamy avocado sauce rich in calcium and healthy fats, this is a dish your taste buds will love.

ZUCCHINI NOODLES

2 large zucchini (about 22 ounces)

1 tablespoon extra-virgin olive oil

2 cloves garlic, minced

1 large red bell pepper, thinly sliced and cut into 1-inch pieces

DRESSING

1 tablespoon extra-virgin olive oil

1 large avocado

¼ cup nonfat (0%) plain Greek yogurt

2 teaspoons fresh lemon juice

2 cloves garlic, minced

2 teaspoons dried basil

Salt and freshly ground black pepper (optional)

SALAD

2 cups frozen shelled edamame

1 cup cherry tomatoes, halved

1 (15-ounce) can black beans, rinsed and drained

3 tablespoons finely chopped chives

TIP: A handheld type of spiralizer is all that is needed for this recipe to keep prep time minimal and efficient. You can find them for less than $10.

1. Make the zucchini noodles: Cut off the ends of the zucchini and spiralize (see Tip). Set the zucchini noodles in a large bowl lined with paper towels to absorb the excess moisture.

2. In a large sauté pan, heat the olive oil over medium-high heat. Add the garlic, bell pepper, and spiralized zucchini. Cook until the vegetables are tender, being careful not to overcook, 6 to 8 minutes.

3. Meanwhile, prepare the dressing: In a blender or food processor, combine the olive oil, avocado, Greek yogurt, ¼ cup water, the lemon juice, garlic, basil, and salt and pepper, if desired, and blend until smooth.

4. Prepare the salad: Place the edamame in a microwave-safe dish, add 1 to 2 tablespoons water, and cook on high until tender, 3 to 5 minutes. Drain and transfer to a large bowl.

5. Add to the bowl the zucchini noodle mixture, the cherry tomatoes, black beans, and chives. Drizzle with the avocado dressing and mix to combine.

6. Portion onto 6 plates.

PER SERVING: Calories: 259; Total fat: 13 g; Saturated fat: 2 g; Cholesterol: <1 mg; Sodium: 27 mg; Potassium: 553 mg; Total carbohydrates: 26 g; Fiber: 10 g; Sugars: 3 g; Protein: 16 g

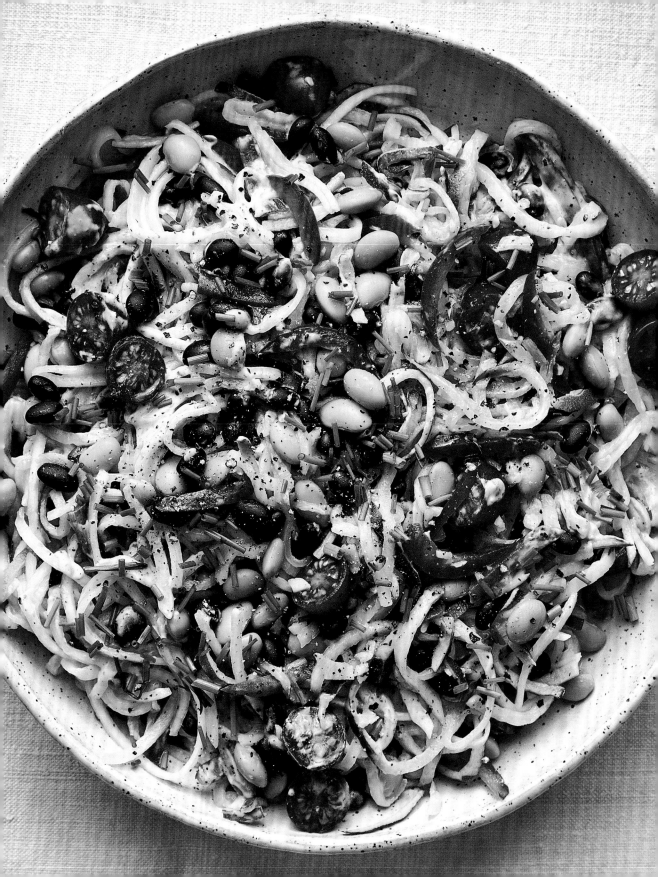

Grilled Turkey and Avocado Salad

Skinless turkey breast is one of the leanest meats available and is an excellent source of high-quality protein. Turkey is rich in heart-healthy B vitamins and contains an abundance of minerals, including immune-boosting zinc. And best of all, turkey breast is very low in calories. Featured in this quick and fiber-rich salad, turkey breast is quickly sautéed on the stovetop and mixed with creamy, satiating seared avocado and fresh vegetables to create a tasty, meal-size salad.

1 tablespoon extra-virgin olive oil, plus more (optional) for drizzling

1 pound turkey breast cutlets (such as Honeysuckle White; see Tip, page 158), cut into 1-inch pieces

2 firm-ripe avocados

8 cups mixed baby greens

1 small red onion, thinly sliced

1 large tomato, coarsely chopped

¼ cup sunflower seeds

¼ cup chopped fresh cilantro

Salt and freshly ground black pepper (optional)

1. On a grill pan or in a large nonstick skillet, heat the olive oil over medium-high heat. Add the turkey breast pieces and cook, stirring constantly, until no longer pink inside, about 10 minutes. Remove from the pan and set aside.

2. Peel, pit, and quarter the avocados. Coat with olive oil cooking spray. Grill in the grill pan or sear in the skillet until lightly browned, 1 to 2 minutes.

3. To serve, portion the salad greens, turkey, avocado, red onion, tomato, sunflower seeds, and cilantro onto 4 serving plates. Sprinkle with salt and pepper and drizzle with additional olive oil, if desired.

TIP: Turkey breast contains the amino acid tryptophan, which is famous for making you sleepy after a Thanksgiving meal. Tryptophan is essential to the production of serotonin, a neurotransmitter, which has a calming effect. Next time you are feeling stressed, consider preparing yourself a turkey salad.

PER SERVING: Calories: 370; Total fat: 21 g; Saturated fat: 3 g; Cholesterol: 70 mg; Sodium: 137 mg; Potassium: 627 mg; Total carbohydrates: 17 g; Fiber: 10 g; Sugars: 1 g; Protein: 33 g

Crunchy Thai Peanut-Edamame Power Salad

Edamame are green soybeans and are loaded with protein, fiber, phytochemicals, and cholesterol-fighting heart-healthy nutrients. A complete plant protein, edamame are a firm, chewy bean much like a lima bean, so they work well in a variety of dishes. Easy to locate fresh or in the freezer section, with their higher protein content, edamame are a good choice for meatless meals. Tossed with a mix of crunchy, nutrient-rich vegetables and a creamy peanut dressing, this salad makes a light lunch, or you can pair it with grilled fish or chicken.

SALAD

1 (16-ounce) package frozen shelled edamame (green soybeans), thawed

4 medium radishes, thinly sliced

1 cup shredded carrots

2 cups thinly sliced red cabbage (see Tips)

2 cups thinly sliced napa cabbage

1 red bell pepper, thinly sliced

½ cup loosely packed chopped fresh cilantro

THAI PEANUT DRESSING

¼ cup unsalted creamy peanut butter

2 tablespoons unseasoned rice vinegar

2 tablespoons fresh lime juice

1 teaspoon reduced-sodium soy sauce (see Tips)

1 tablespoon honey

1-inch piece fresh ginger, peeled and coarsely chopped

½ teaspoon hot sauce

Very hot water

1. Prepare the salad: Cook the edamame according to the package directions, omitting the salt. Cool under running cold water and drain well.

2. In a large bowl, toss together the edamame, radishes, carrots, red cabbage, napa cabbage, bell pepper, and cilantro.

3. Make the Thai peanut dressing: In a small bowl, whisk together the peanut butter, rice vinegar, lime juice, soy sauce, honey, ginger, and hot sauce. Add very hot water 1 tablespoon at a time until the dressing is pourable.

4. Drizzle the peanut dressing over the edamame/vegetable mixture and toss to thoroughly coat.

TIPS: If you have a hard time finding red cabbage, substitute angel hair cabbage/coleslaw.

To reduce the sodium content of the dressing further, omit the soy sauce and replace it with 1 tablespoon balsamic vinegar.

PER SERVING: Calories: 223; Total fat: 10 g; Saturated fat: 1 g; Cholesterol: 0 mg; Sodium: 101 mg; Potassium: 328 mg; Total carbohydrates: 22 g; Fiber: 7 g; Sugars: 8 g; Protein: 12 g

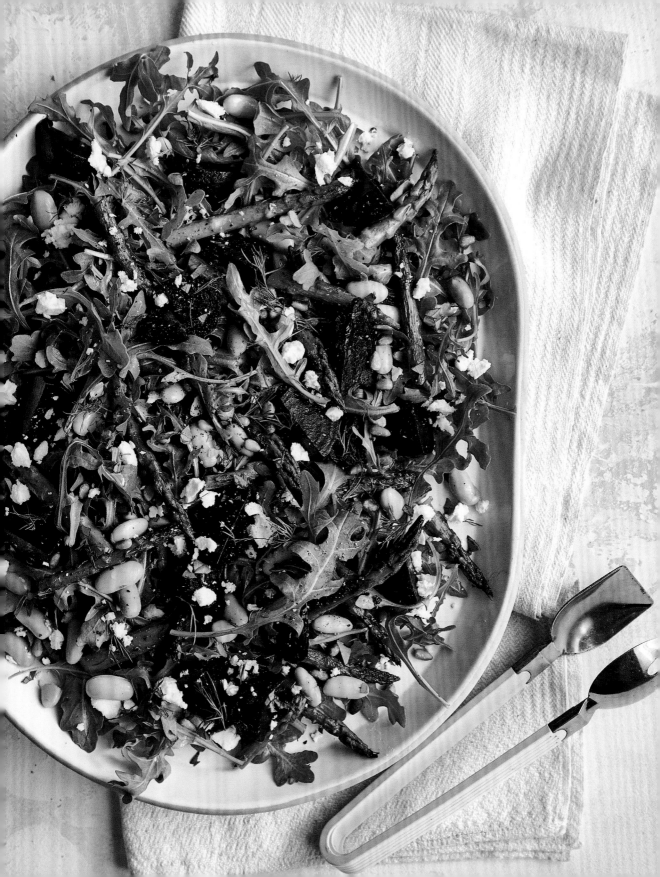

Roasted Asparagus, Beet, and Cannellini Bean Salad

Beets, beans, and asparagus are three of the best foods you can eat for lowering blood pressure and losing weight. Beets are rich in plant nitrates, which relax blood vessels, asparagus acts as a natural diuretic, and beans provide energy-sustaining and hunger-squashing protein and fiber. Served on top of peppery baby arugula, the flavors come together in perfect harmony.

4 medium beets (about 1 pound)

2 cloves garlic, peeled but whole

2 tablespoons extra-virgin olive oil

Salt and freshly ground black pepper

½ pound asparagus, tough ends trimmed

1 (15-ounce) can cannellini beans, rinsed and drained

⅓ cup pine nuts

2 tablespoons finely chopped fresh basil

2 tablespoons finely chopped fresh dill

8 cups baby arugula

2 tablespoons crumbled low-fat feta cheese

1 lemon, halved

1. Preheat the oven to 425°F.

2. Set the beets and garlic on a large piece of foil and drizzle with 1 tablespoon of the olive oil, sprinkle with a pinch of salt and black pepper and a splash of water. Fold the foil up into a pouch and seal the edges. Transfer to the oven and roast until the beets are easily pierced with a knife, 35 to 40 minutes.

3. Meanwhile, place the asparagus on a foil-lined baking sheet and drizzle with the remaining 1 tablespoon olive oil, then rub each stalk with your hands to evenly coat with oil. Sprinkle with salt and black pepper, if desired.

4. When the beets have cooked for about 20 minutes, place the asparagus in the oven and roast until the toughest parts of the stalks are tender and the leafy tips are starting to get crispy, 12 to 15 minutes.

5. While the vegetables roast, in a medium bowl, toss together the beans, pine nuts, basil, and dill.

6. Remove the beets and asparagus from the oven and allow to cool slightly. Remove the skins from the beets with a paper towel or gloves and discard. Cut the beets into ½-inch pieces. Slice the roasted garlic thinly and cut each asparagus stalk into 4 or 5 pieces.

7. Add the beets, garlic, and asparagus to the bean mixture and toss to combine.

8. To serve, top each plate with 2 cups arugula and ½ tablespoon feta and squeeze fresh lemon on top.

TIP: Feta cheese is very high in sodium, but it has an intense flavor so you only need a very small amount to make a recipe pop.

PER SERVING: Calories: 318; Total fat: 15 g; Saturated fat: 2 g; Cholesterol: 2 mg; Sodium: 117 mg; Potassium: 286 mg; Total carbohydrates: 36 g; Fiber: 9 g; Sugars: 17 g; Protein: 12 g

Farmers' Market Chickpea Salad

This fresh and tasty salad makes use of the bounty of seasonal produce at its national peak in warmer months. Green beans are a nutrient-dense, low-calorie choice rich in beta-carotene, vitamins C, K, B$_6$, and folate, and the minerals calcium, potassium, and iron. Blanching them quickly means they remain crisp and tender with nutrients intact. Fiber- and protein-rich chickpeas, cucumbers, tomatoes, fresh herbs, and inflammation-reducing walnuts round out this filling salad that is colorful and delicious.

1 pound green beans, ends trimmed

1 (15-ounce) can chickpeas, rinsed and drained

2 cups cherry tomatoes, halved

1 cup Persian (mini) cucumber slices

¼ cup chopped fresh flat-leaf parsley

2 tablespoons chopped fresh mint or 1 teaspoon dried

1 tablespoon extra-virgin olive oil

¼ cup chopped walnuts

1 lemon, halved

Salt and freshly ground black pepper (optional)

TIP: This salad also makes a great appetizer or side dish for grilled chicken or fish, and can be divided into 4 or 6 servings, depending on your needs.

1. Bring a large pot of water to a boil over high heat. Add the beans and blanch until bright green and crisp-tender, 3 to 5 minutes. Immediately rinse with cold water to stop the cooking.

2. Meanwhile, in a medium bowl, combine the chickpeas, tomatoes, cucumber, parsley, mint, olive oil, and walnuts and toss to combine.

3. To serve, divide the green beans between 2 serving plates and top each with half of the chickpea mixture. Top each with a squeeze of fresh lemon. If desired, season with salt and pepper.

PER SERVING: Calories: 493; Total fat: 21 g; Saturated fat: 2 g; Cholesterol: 0 mg; Sodium: 40 mg; Potassium: 1,300 mg; Total carbohydrates: 65 g; Fiber: 22 g; Sugars: 14 g; Protein: 19 g

Curried Roasted Cauliflower and Lentil Salad

Very low in calories and extremely versatile, cauliflower boasts a host of health benefits including an abundance of antioxidants, vitamins, and minerals that fight inflammation and reduce the risk for heart disease, diabetes, and certain cancers. This recipe roasts the cauliflower with Indian-inspired seasonings and couples it with protein- and fiber-rich lentils to create a filling and satiating salad that tastes great warm, at room temperature, or even cold.

1 head cauliflower, cut into florets

1 small red onion, thinly sliced into half-moons

2 tablespoons extra-virgin olive oil

1 teaspoon ground turmeric

1 teaspoon curry powder

½ teaspoon ground ginger

Pinch of salt

1 cup brown lentils, rinsed

1 bay leaf

¼ cup golden raisins

¾ cup sliced almonds

8 cups mixed baby greens

1 lemon, halved

½ cup loosely packed cilantro leaves

TIP: Lentils are an outstanding choice for a DASH weight-loss plan. They are a legume (like beans), but are higher in protein and fiber and lower in calories than most beans. They are also very satiating and help regulate blood-sugar levels because they are composed of slow-digesting complex carbohydrates.

1. Preheat the oven to 400°F. Line a rimmed baking sheet with foil or parchment.

2. In a large bowl, toss the cauliflower florets and sliced onion with the olive oil, turmeric, curry powder, ginger, and salt. Spread in an even layer on the prepared baking sheet. Bake until the cauliflower and onions are tender and lightly browned, about 25 minutes.

3. Meanwhile, in a medium saucepan, combine the lentils and bay leaf and add enough water to cover by 1 inch (about 2 cups). Bring to a boil, reduce the heat, and simmer uncovered until the lentils are tender but not mushy, 16 to 20 minutes.

4. Drain the lentils and discard the bay leaf. Set aside to cool.

5. When everything is cooled, in a medium bowl, toss together the roasted cauliflower and onions, lentils, raisins, and almonds.

6. To assemble the salads, place 2 cups greens on each of 4 serving plates. Divide the cauliflower/lentil mixture among the plates, and top with a squeeze of fresh lemon and the cilantro.

PER SERVING: Calories: 437; Total fat: 20 g; Saturated fat: 2 g; Cholesterol: 0 mg; Sodium: 141 mg; Potassium: 1,154 mg; Total carbohydrates: 53 g; Fiber: 23 g; Sugars: 12 g; Protein: 22 g

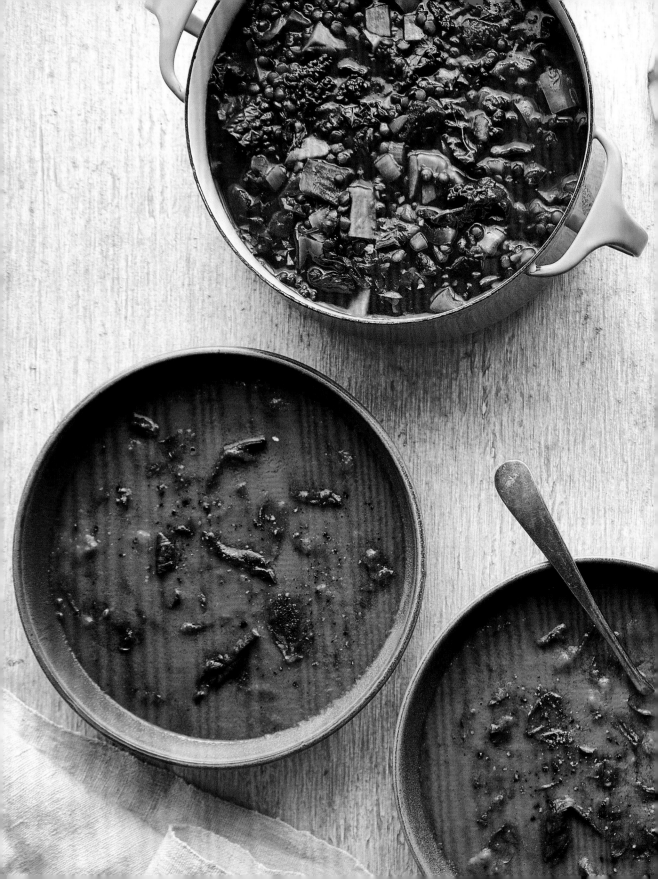

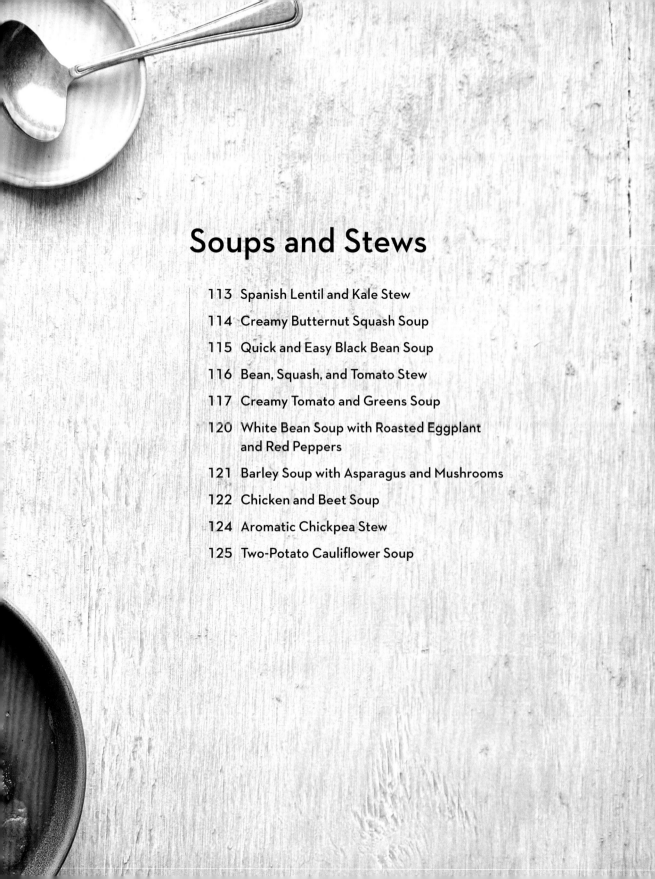

Soups and Stews

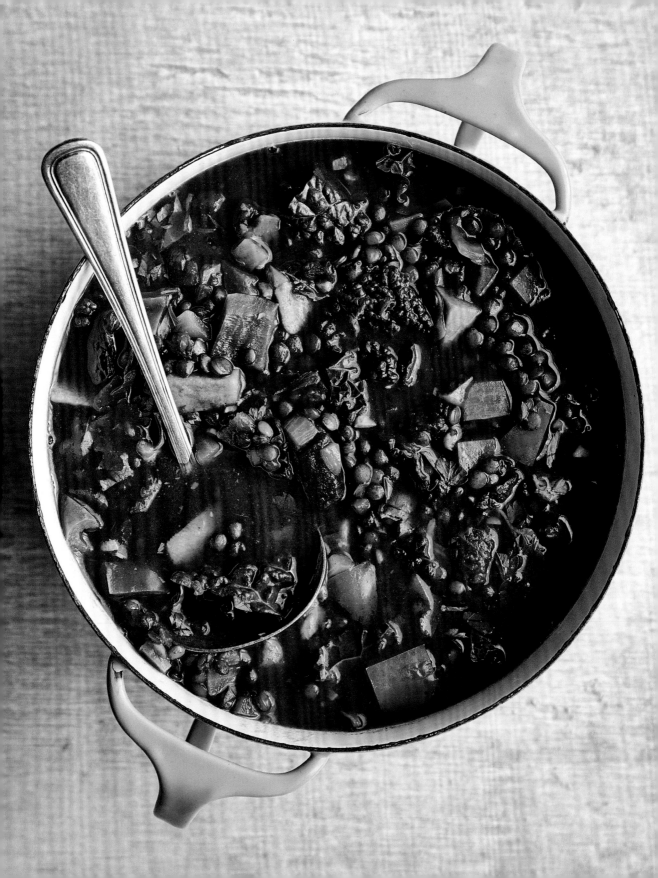

Spanish Lentil and Kale Stew

This hearty and nutritious lentil and kale stew uses spices common to Spanish cooking, including smoked paprika, rosemary, cayenne, and parsley. Budget friendly and made using pantry staples, this comforting and delicious stew is full of plant protein, fiber, vitamins, and minerals, while being low in calories. Serve with crusty whole-grain bread topped with avocado and tomato slices for a warm and earthy meatless meal.

1 tablespoon extra-virgin olive oil

1 medium red onion, finely diced

1 medium green bell pepper, chopped

3 cloves garlic, minced

5 cups low-sodium vegetable broth

1 bay leaf

1¼ cups brown or green lentils, rinsed

1 medium carrot, chopped

1 medium sweet potato, peeled and cubed

1 (14.5-ounce) can no-salt-added diced tomatoes, undrained

1½ teaspoons smoked paprika

1 teaspoon ground rosemary

¼ teaspoon cayenne pepper

½ cup frozen chopped kale, thawed and squeezed dry (½ of a 10-ounce package)

½ cup chopped fresh parsley

1 tablespoon cooking sherry

Salt and freshly ground black pepper (optional)

1. In a large pot or Dutch oven, heat the olive oil over medium heat. Add the onion and bell pepper and cook until softened, 4 to 5 minutes. Add the garlic and cook until fragrant, 2 to 3 minutes.

2. Add the broth, bay leaf, lentils, carrot, sweet potato, diced tomatoes and their juices, paprika, rosemary, and cayenne. Bring to a boil, then cover and let simmer over medium-low heat until the lentils and vegetables are tender, 25 to 30 minutes.

3. Add the kale, parsley, cooking sherry, and salt and pepper, if desired, and continue cooking for 10 minutes to thicken (see Tip) the stew.

4. Remove the bay leaf and serve.

TIP: This soup can be served thick or thin. Add more water if you want it to be more of a soup than a stew. It also thickens as it cools.

PER SERVING: Calories: 226; Total fat: 3 g; Saturated fat: <1 g; Cholesterol: 0 mg; Sodium: 148 mg; Potassium: 526 mg; Total carbohydrates: 39 g; Fiber: 14 g; Sugars: 9 g; Protein: 12 g

Creamy Butternut Squash Soup

Just 1 cooked cup of creamy butternut squash provides 500 milligrams of heart-healthy potassium, 160 percent of the RDA for vitamin A, 7 grams of dietary fiber, along with numerous other nutrients for less than 100 calories. Roasted with carrot and apple, pureed until silky smooth, and mixed with creamy Greek yogurt, this soup may become a regular on your menu.

1 (12-ounce) package cubed peeled butternut squash

1 medium carrot, sliced

1 Granny Smith apple, cubed

1 teaspoon ground cinnamon

½ teaspoon ground ginger

½ teaspoon ground turmeric

½ teaspoon ground nutmeg

2 tablespoons extra-virgin olive oil

1 medium onion, chopped

3 cloves garlic, sliced

4 cups low-sodium vegetable broth

⅔ cup nonfat (0%) plain Greek yogurt

Salt and freshly ground black pepper (optional)

TIP: Butternut squash isn't just for savory dishes. It's also a great addition to smoothies. Frozen butternut squash pairs well with raspberries, peanut butter, frozen banana, cashew milk, and vanilla plant protein.

1. Preheat the oven to 400°F. Line a rimmed baking sheet with foil.

2. In a medium bowl, combine the butternut squash, carrot, apple, cinnamon, ginger, turmeric, nutmeg, and 1 tablespoon of the olive oil and toss to coat. Spread in an even layer on the baking sheet and roast until softened, 10 to 12 minutes.

3. In a large pot or Dutch oven, heat the remaining 1 tablespoon olive oil over medium-high heat. Add the onion and garlic and cook until tender, 4 to 5 minutes.

4. Add the roasted squash mixture and cook 5 minutes, until heated through, stirring constantly to avoid sticking. Add the broth and simmer for 30 minutes.

5. Remove from the heat and stir in the yogurt. Using an immersion blender, puree the soup until smooth (or transfer in batches to a blender or food processor, puree until smooth, and return to the pot). Stir in salt and pepper, if desired, and simmer gently for 5 minutes.

6. Ladle soup into 6 bowls and serve.

PER SERVING: Calories: 205; Total fat: 7 g; Saturated fat: 1 g; Cholesterol: 2 mg; Sodium: 178 mg; Potassium: 684 mg; Total carbohydrates: 32 g; Fiber: 8 g; Sugars: 13 g; Protein: 6 g

Quick and Easy Black Bean Soup

This soup recipe is super quick and will remind you how easy and uncomplicated cooking can be. Additionally, broth-based soups are ideal for a weight-loss plan because they are full of fiber and very filling, leading you to eat less throughout the day. Black beans are high in blood-pressure-lowering potassium, B vitamins, fiber, and protein as well as disease-reducing phytochemicals. Simple, tasty, nutritious, and satisfying, this recipe comes together in less than 20 minutes and can be made with pantry staples.

2 (15-ounce) cans black beans, rinsed and drained

1 tablespoon extra-virgin olive oil

1 medium onion, diced

4 cloves garlic, minced

2 (14.5-ounce) cans no-salt-added (see Tip) fire-roasted tomatoes

1 cup low-sodium vegetable broth, plus more as needed

1 teaspoon ground cumin

½ teaspoon chili powder

1 tablespoon fresh lime juice

Salt and freshly ground black pepper (optional)

½ cup chopped fresh cilantro

TIP: If you are watching your sodium intake, be conscious of the amount of sodium in the canned ingredients you use. Many canned foods are sold in low-sodium or no-salt-added versions, so choose these if possible. Keep in mind that just 1 teaspoon table salt has almost 2,400 mg of sodium, which is your entire day's allowance.

1. In a food processor or blender, pulse half of the black beans until thickened but not fully pureed.

2. In a large pot or Dutch oven, heat the olive oil over medium-high heat. Add the onion and garlic and sauté until softened and lightly browned, 4 to 5 minutes.

3. Stir in the processed black beans, the remaining whole black beans, the tomatoes, broth, cumin, and chili powder. Bring to a simmer and cook for 10 to 15 minutes, until thickened. If the soup is too thick, add additional broth; if it is too thin, puree 1 to 2 cups of the soup in a blender and return it to the pot (or use an immersion blender to puree directly in the pot until your desired consistency is reached).

4. Remove from the heat and stir in the lime juice. Season with salt and pepper, if desired. Portion into 4 serving bowls and top with the cilantro.

PER SERVING: Calories: 262; Total fat: 4 g; Saturated fat: <1 g; Cholesterol: 0 mg; Sodium: 59 mg; Potassium: 55 mg; Total carbohydrates: 44 g; Fiber: 11 g; Sugars: 9 g; Protein: 13 g

Bean, Squash, and Tomato Stew

This is a simple, fiber- and plant protein–rich dish that you can put together in a snap using pantry ingredients. Seasoned with Middle Eastern spices, this recipe has a thick, chili-like consistency that is filling and satisfying. This stew is full of potassium, vitamin C, and fiber, but feel free to substitute your favorite vegetables or add more for increased nutrition.

2 tablespoons extra-virgin olive oil

1 small red onion, thinly sliced

5 cups zucchini, about 2 large zucchini, chopped

2 celery stalks, sliced

4 cloves garlic, sliced

1 (14.5-ounce) can no-salt-added diced tomatoes, undrained

1 teaspoon ground coriander

1 teaspoon ground cumin

½ teaspoon ground cinnamon

Salt and freshly ground black pepper (optional)

1 (15-ounce) can red beans, rinsed and drained

¼ cup chopped fresh cilantro

1. In a large saucepan, heat the olive oil over medium-low heat. Add the onion, zucchini, and celery and cook until soft and translucent, 8 to 10 minutes. Add the garlic and cook for 1 minute.

2. Add the tomatoes and their juices, the coriander, cumin, cinnamon, and salt and pepper, if desired. Bring to a boil and simmer for 10 minutes.

3. Add the beans and 2 cups water, cover, and simmer for another 15 to 20 minutes to thicken the stew and blend the flavors.

4. Serve garnished with fresh cilantro.

PER SERVING: Calories: 442; Total fat: 14 g; Saturated fat: 2 g; Cholesterol: 0 mg; Sodium: 94 mg; Potassium: 1,404 mg; Total carbohydrates: 65 g; Fiber: 19 g; Sugars: 18 g; Protein: 17 g

TIP: Zucchini is widely available year-round and is extremely versatile, low in calories, and a good source of potassium. One cup of slices has a mere 19 calories.

Creamy Tomato and Greens Soup

Budget friendly and delicious, this creamy potassium- and calcium-rich tomato and greens soup is so simple to make using fresh ingredients, yet so decadent tasting you won't believe how healthy it is. Starting with fresh tomatoes and cooking them down releases their sweet flavors, which is complemented by the hearty, rich flavors of spinach. Serve this with a healthy homemade grilled cheese sandwich for a cozy, comforting meal.

2 tablespoons extra-virgin olive oil

1 medium red onion, diced

3 cloves garlic, minced

12 Roma (plum) tomatoes, seeded and diced

1 tablespoon tomato paste

1 cup fresh basil leaves

½ teaspoon dried thyme

3 cups low-sodium vegetable broth, plus more as needed

¼ teaspoon freshly ground black pepper

1 cup frozen spinach, thawed

½ cup nonfat (0%) plain Greek yogurt (see Tip)

TIP: You can make this vegan by replacing the Greek yogurt with pureed silken tofu, almond milk, or a nondairy yogurt.

1. In a large soup pot or Dutch oven, heat the olive oil over medium heat. Add the onion and sauté until translucent, 5 to 7 minutes.

2. Add the garlic and cook for 1 minute. Add the tomatoes, tomato paste, basil, thyme, broth, and black pepper and stir well. Bring the soup to a boil, then reduce the heat and simmer, uncovered, until the tomatoes are very tender, about 30 minutes.

3. Using an immersion blender, puree the soup until smooth (or transfer in batches to a blender or food processor and puree until smooth, returning the soup to the pot).

4. Add the spinach and stir and cook for 4 to 5 minutes, until warmed through.

5. Remove from the heat and allow to cool slightly before stirring in the Greek yogurt (to avoid curdling). This soup has a fairly thick consistency, so if you like a thinner soup, simply add a bit more broth.

PER SERVING: Calories: 161; Total fat: 8 g; Saturated fat: 1 g; Cholesterol: 1 mg; Sodium: 221 mg; Potassium: 789 mg; Total carbohydrates: 20 g; Fiber: 6 g; Sugars: 5 g; Protein: 7 g

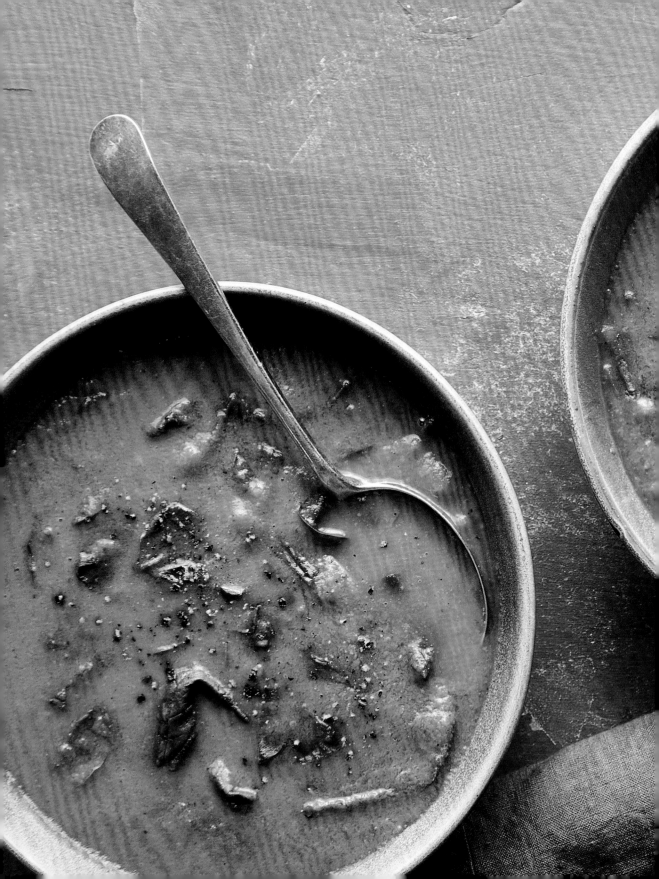

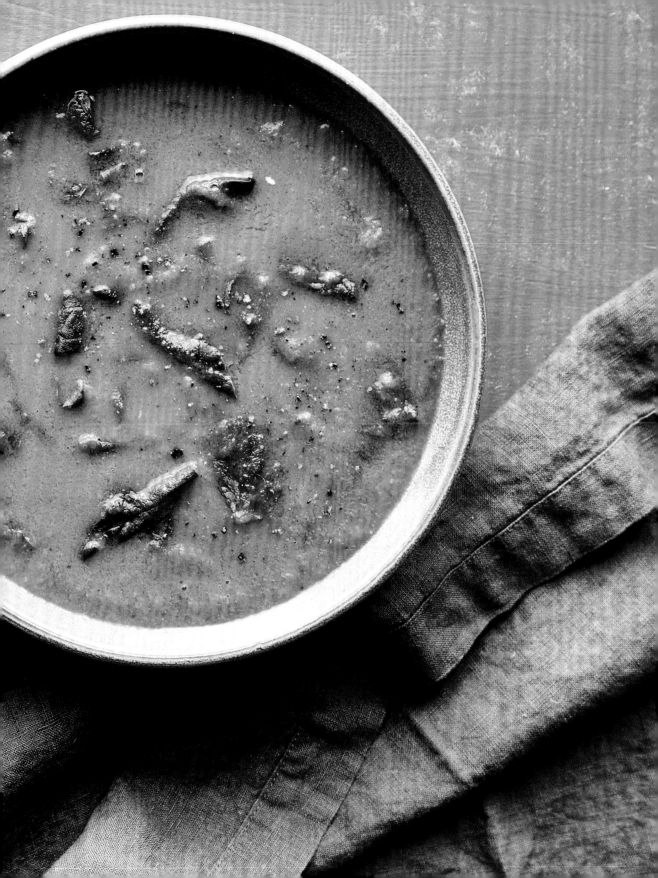

White Bean Soup with Roasted Eggplant and Red Peppers

Healthy eating isn't about feeling deprived or miserable, and this flavorful, creamy, and satisfying soup is a testament to that. Eggplant is high in dietary fiber and potassium and very low in calories (because it is 90 percent water), and red bell peppers boast numerous antioxidants, vitamins, and minerals. Roasting both of these vegetables brings out their natural sweetness. With the addition of white beans, this protein-packed, delicious, and creamy soup makes a filling meal.

2 medium red bell peppers, halved

1 medium eggplant (about 1¼ pounds), unpeeled, halved lengthwise (see Tip)

1 tablespoon extra-virgin olive oil

1 large onion, chopped

4 cloves garlic, minced

1½ cups low-sodium vegetable broth

2 (15-ounce) cans white beans, rinsed and drained

2 teaspoons dried thyme

Salt and freshly ground black pepper (optional)

1. Preheat the broiler. Line a rimmed baking sheet with foil.

2. Place the bell peppers and eggplant halves cut side down on the baking sheet, pressing them down to make them as flat as possible.

3. Broil until the skins are blackened on all sides, 10 to 15 minutes. Remove from the oven and place in a covered container or paper bag or wrap in foil to steam for a few minutes.

4. Meanwhile, in a large pot, heat the olive oil over medium-high heat. Add the onion and garlic and sauté until softened and fragrant, 4 to 5 minutes. Add the broth, beans, and thyme and continue cooking while you peel the eggplant and peppers.

5. When the roasted vegetables are cool enough to handle, scoop the flesh from the eggplant and add to the pot (discard the skin). Remove the charred outer skin from the bell peppers and add the peppers to the pot. Bring the soup to a simmer over medium-low heat and cook for 10 minutes.

6. Using an immersion blender, puree the soup until smooth (or transfer in batches to a blender or food processor and puree until smooth).

7. Taste and add salt and pepper, if desired, and simmer on low for 10 minutes to allow the flavors to develop.

TIP: Today's eggplant is not as bitter as it was years ago because of changes in how it is grown. However, if you are concerned with bitterness, salt the flesh and let it sit for 10 minutes, then squeeze or press the salt off before using.

PER SERVING: Calories: 312; Total fat: 4 g; Saturated fat: <1 g; Cholesterol: 0 mg; Sodium: 67 mg; Potassium: 1,248 mg; Total carbohydrates: 56 g; Fiber: 14 g; Sugars: 7 g; Protein: 15 g

Barley Soup with Asparagus and Mushrooms

Barley is one of the best grains to eat for reducing cholesterol due to its high content of beta-glucan, a type of soluble fiber that binds to cholesterol for removal from the body. By adding asparagus (a natural diuretic), calcium-rich greens, and white beans for appetite control, I've amped up the blood-pressure-lowering and weight-loss powers of this soup. While the least processed form of barley, hulled, has the highest fiber content, it is hard to find and takes longer to cook. For cooking ease, use pearl barley and know that you will still receive health benefits. Enjoy this delicious bowl of comfort with crusty whole-grain bread.

2 tablespoons extra-virgin olive oil

1 clove garlic, minced

1 medium onion, chopped

1 medium carrot, diced

1 small bunch asparagus, tough ends trimmed, cut into 1- to 2-inch pieces

10 ounces mushrooms, sliced

¾ cup pearl barley (or hulled barley, soaked overnight)

4 cups low-sodium vegetable broth

2 bay leaves

1 teaspoon dried marjoram

1 teaspoon sweet paprika

½ teaspoon ground turmeric

1 (15-ounce) can white beans, rinsed and drained

4 leaves kale, midribs removed, thinly sliced

3 tablespoons cooking sherry

Freshly ground black pepper (optional)

¼ cup minced fresh parsley

1. In a large soup pot, heat the olive oil over medium heat. Add the garlic, onion, and carrot and cook, stirring occasionally, until the vegetables have softened, 8 to 10 minutes.

2. Add the asparagus and mushrooms, stir well, and continue to cook for another 5 minutes.

3. Add the barley, broth, bay leaves, marjoram, paprika, and turmeric and bring to a boil. Reduce the heat to low, cover, and simmer until the barley is tender and plumps up, 30 to 40 minutes for pearl barley, 60 minutes for hulled barley. If the soup seems too thick at any point, add more water, ½ cup at a time.

4. When the barley is tender, stir in the beans, kale, and sherry and continue to cook for 10 minutes.

5. Season with pepper, if desired, and stir in the parsley before serving.

TIP: Soups freeze well and can be a lifesaver on those hectic days when you are too tired to cook. Consider making it a part of your routine to cook a pot of soup on the weekends and freeze a couple of servings. After a few weeks of doing this, you will have a variety on hand to choose from.

PER SERVING: Calories: 372; Total fat: 8 g; Saturated fat: 1 g; Cholesterol: 0 mg; Sodium: 173 mg; Potassium: 964 mg; Total carbohydrates: 69 g; Fiber: 15 g; Sugars: 7 g; Protein: 14 g

Chicken and Beet Soup

This vibrantly colored soup has everything you need for a meal that satisfies your appetite for a few calories while providing your heart with blood-pressure-lowering nutrients. The beets and vegetables gently flavor the broth while they simmer, adding a subtle sweetness. Don't skip the fresh dill, as it really adds to the flavor of the soup. A taste sensation, this soup would also make a great first course.

1 tablespoon extra-virgin olive oil

¾ pound boneless, skinless chicken breasts, cut into 1-inch pieces

1 medium onion, diced

1 clove garlic, minced

2 cups low-sodium chicken broth

1 pound beets, peeled and grated (about 2½ cups; see Tip)

3 medium carrots, cut into ¼-inch-thick slices (2 cups)

1 teaspoon dried tarragon

1 teaspoon dried dill

¼ cup chopped fresh dill

Freshly ground black pepper

1. In a large nonstick Dutch oven or soup pot, heat the olive oil over medium-high until hot. Add the chicken, onion, and garlic and cook until the chicken is no longer pink, 5 to 7 minutes.

2. Add the broth, 2 cups water, the beets, carrots, tarragon, and dried dill and mix well. Bring to a boil, then reduce the heat, cover, and simmer until the vegetables are very tender, 15 to 20 minutes. Stir in the fresh dill and season to taste with black pepper.

PER SERVING: Calories: 207; Total fat: 6 g; Saturated fat: <1 g; Cholesterol: 49 mg; Sodium: 303 mg; Potassium: 634 mg; Total carbohydrates: 20 g; Fiber: 5 g; Sugars: 12 g; Protein: 21 g

TIP: For easy cleanup, peel and grate the beets in the sink. A box grater works well or a food processor with a shredding blade may be a timesaver.

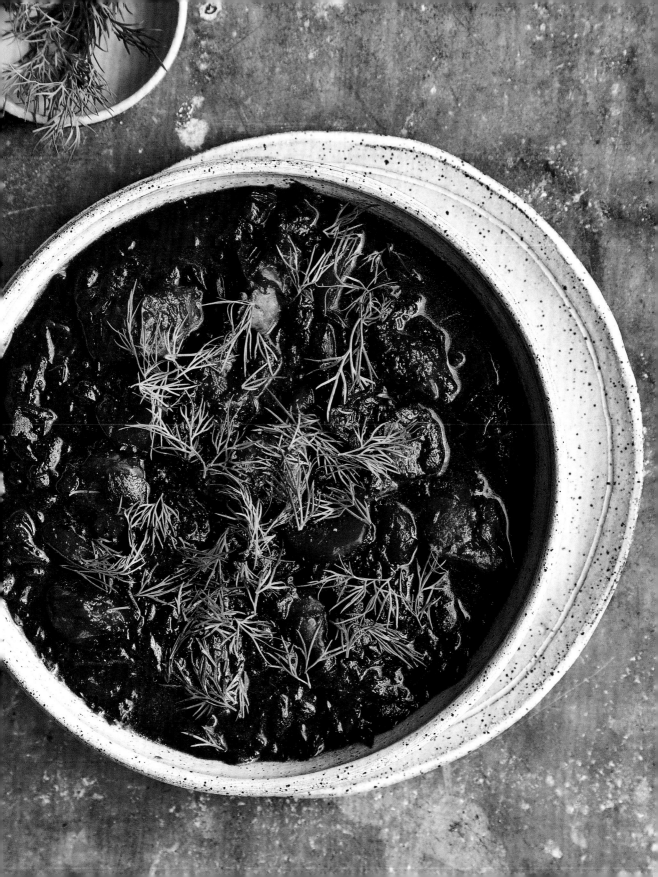

Aromatic Chickpea Stew

Made with simple pantry ingredients, this deeply flavored and aromatic stew is seasoned with toasted cumin and earthy, antioxidant-rich spices—including garam masala, paprika, and turmeric—and is full of plant protein, fiber, potassium, and calcium. Serve over Herbed Cauliflower and Broccoli Rice (page 211) for a filling meal that keeps calories in check.

1 tablespoon extra-virgin olive oil

2 teaspoons cumin seeds

1 medium red onion, chopped

4 cloves garlic, minced

1 medium red bell pepper, chopped

2 medium tomatoes, chopped

1 medium carrot, diced

1 medium zucchini, sliced

1 teaspoon ground coriander

1 teaspoon garam masala (see Tip)

1 teaspoon sweet paprika

1 teaspoon ground turmeric

2 (15-ounce) cans chickpeas, rinsed and drained

1 tablespoon tomato paste

10 ounces frozen spinach, thawed

Salt and freshly ground black pepper (optional)

Pinch of cayenne pepper (optional)

2 tablespoons finely chopped fresh cilantro

1. In a large saucepan, heat the olive oil over medium-high heat. Add the cumin seeds and cook for 10 seconds. Add the onion and garlic and cook until translucent, 3 minutes.

2. Add the bell pepper, tomatoes, carrot, and zucchini and cook, stirring until starting to soften, 5 to 6 minutes.

3. Add the coriander, garam masala, paprika, and turmeric and cook, stirring, for 1 minute.

4. Stir in 2 cups water, the chickpeas, tomato paste, and spinach and bring to a boil. Reduce the heat to low, cover, and simmer until the vegetables are tender, the sauce has thickened slightly, and the flavors have melded, 15 to 20 minutes.

5. Remove from the heat, taste, and season with salt, pepper, and cayenne, if desired. Serve garnished with the cilantro.

TIP: Garam masala is a spice blend used in Indian cooking. You can make your own by mixing together 1 tablespoon ground cumin, 1½ teaspoons ground coriander, 1½ teaspoons ground cardamom, 1½ teaspoons ground black pepper, 1 teaspoon ground cinnamon, ½ teaspoon ground cloves, and ½ teaspoon ground nutmeg.

PER SERVING: Calories: 309; Total fat: 7 g; Saturated fat: <1 g; Cholesterol: 0 mg; Sodium: 134 mg; Potassium: 1,056 mg; Total carbohydrates: 50 g; Fiber: 14 g; Sugars: 10 g; Protein: 15 g

Two-Potato Cauliflower Soup

Not your ordinary potato soup, this recipe combines the buttery taste of Yukon Gold potatoes with the syrupy taste of sweet potatoes, plus an extra dose of creaminess from the addition of cauliflower. Gold potatoes are one of the best sources of dietary potassium and vitamin C, while sweet potatoes are rich in beta-carotene and fiber, as well as other vitamins and minerals. Cauliflower, a nutrient-dense cruciferous vegetable, makes the soup even heartier while keeping calories in check. Serve this with a fresh green salad with beans and veggies for a complete meal.

1 tablespoon extra-virgin olive oil

1 leek, thinly sliced

2 cloves garlic, minced

2 cups cauliflower florets

½ pound sweet potatoes, peeled and chopped

½ pound Yukon Gold potatoes, unpeeled and chopped

3 cups low-sodium vegetable broth

1 cup fat-free milk or plant-based milk

1 teaspoon sweet paprika

½ teaspoon freshly ground black pepper, or more to taste

¼ cup chopped fresh chives (optional)

1. In a large soup pot or saucepan, heat the olive oil over medium heat. Add the leek and cook until softened, 3 to 5 minutes. Add the garlic and cook for 1 minute.

2. Stir in the cauliflower, sweet potatoes, gold potatoes, and broth and bring to a boil. Reduce the heat, cover, and simmer until the vegetables are tender, 15 to 20 minutes.

3. Using an immersion blender, puree the soup until smooth (or transfer in batches to a blender or food processor and puree until smooth, then return to the pot).

4. Stir in the milk, paprika, and black pepper and cook for 3 to 5 minutes more to heat through.

5. Serve topped with fresh chives, if desired.

TIP: Make it a goal to reduce your food waste. For example, if I have a sweet potato that I won't use before it goes bad, I cook it in the microwave, chop it, and freeze it for use in smoothies. Think about how you can make use of fruits and vegetables before discarding.

PER SERVING: Calories: 181; Total fat: 4 g; Saturated fat: <1 g; Cholesterol: 1 mg; Sodium: 182 mg; Potassium: 786 mg; Total carbohydrates: 33 g; Fiber: 6 g; Sugars: 10 g; Protein: 6 g

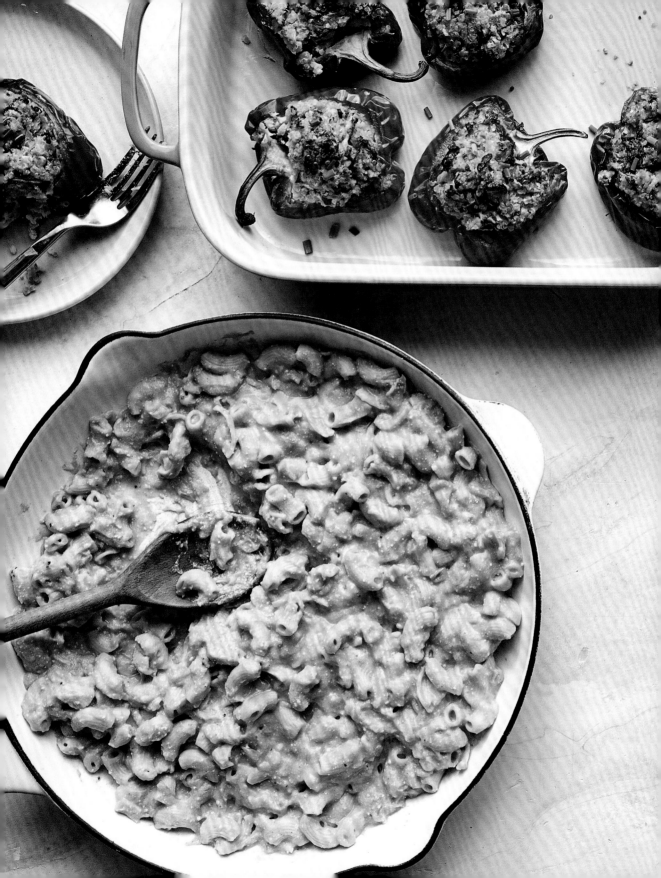

Vegetarian and Vegan Mains

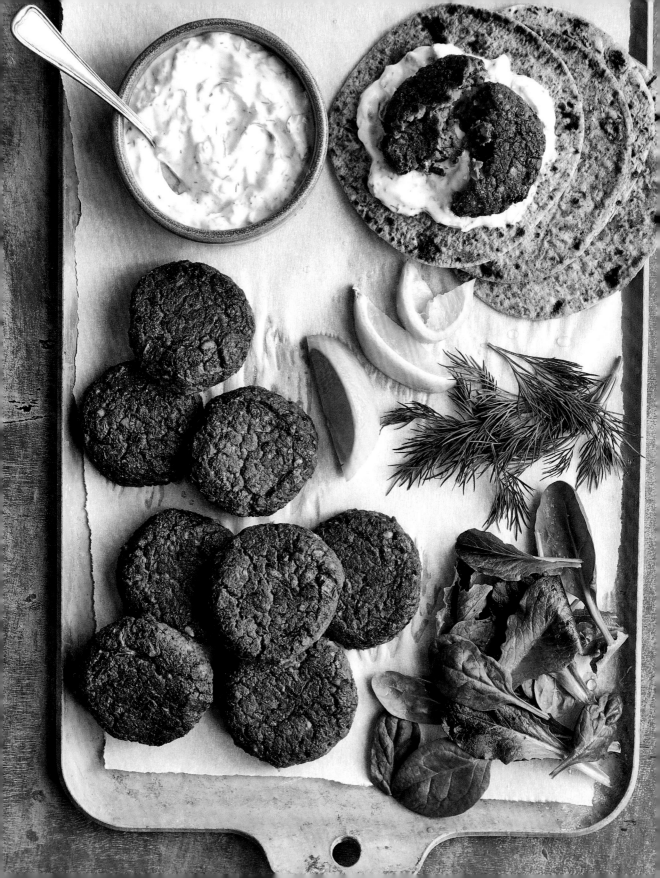

PREP TIME: 15 MINUTES • COOK TIME: 30 MINUTES • SERVES 4

Roasted Red Pepper and Spinach Falafel

Falafel is a traditional Middle Eastern dish of spiced, mashed chickpeas that are formed into small balls and deep-fried. This version lowers the fat and calories by baking the falafel, and boosts the nutrition content by adding rich-tasting roasted red peppers and some spinach for added fiber, vitamins, and minerals. Falafel is something I make often, as it is easy to prepare, easy to customize, freezes well, and is a healthy, filling meal high in plant-powered protein. Serve with a dollop of tahini (sesame paste) or the accompanying tzatziki—where the traditional full-fat regular yogurt is swapped out for protein-rich nonfat (0%) Greek yogurt—and a side of Quinoa Tabbouleh (page 217).

FALAFEL

1 (15-ounce) can chickpeas, rinsed and drained

⅓ cup chopped red onion

4 cloves garlic, coarsely chopped

½ cup packed fresh parsley, destemmed

½ cup jarred roasted red peppers (see Tip), drained

1 cup baby spinach

2 teaspoons ground cumin

2 teaspoons sweet paprika

1 teaspoon ground coriander

1 teaspoon freshly ground black pepper

⅛ teaspoon cayenne pepper

⅛ teaspoon salt

2 teaspoons extra-virgin olive oil

1 tablespoon fresh lemon juice

About ¼ cup chickpea flour (or other flour)

2 tablespoons black or white sesame seeds (optional)

TZATZIKI

½ cup nonfat (0%) plain Greek yogurt

⅓ cup peeled and grated cucumber

1 tablespoon minced fresh dill

1 teaspoon fresh lemon juice

¼ teaspoon minced garlic

1. Make the falafel: Preheat the oven to 375°F. Line a baking sheet with parchment paper.

2. In a food processor, combine the chickpeas, onion, garlic, parsley, roasted red peppers, spinach, cumin, paprika, coriander, black pepper, cayenne, salt, olive oil, and lemon juice. Pulse several times, then blend until fully incorporated but not entirely smooth, as you want a bit of texture.

3. Scoop out the falafel mixture into a large bowl and add the chickpea flour 1 tablespoon at a time until you have a workable dough that isn't too sticky but is still a bit wet.

4. Place the sesame seeds (if using) in a small bowl.

Continued

5. Using a large spoon, measure out portions of the mixture and form into golf ball-size balls (I usually get 12 balls but you can make as many or few as you like). If you are using the optional sesame seeds, roll the balls in the seeds. Place the falafel on the lined baking sheet and flatten them a bit with the palm of your hand.

6. Transfer to the oven and bake until browned, about 30 minutes, turning halfway through.

7. While the falafel are baking, make the tzatziki: In a small bowl, stir together the yogurt, cucumber, dill, lemon juice, and garlic. Refrigerate until ready to use.

8. Serve the falafel with the tzatziki sauce. These also make a great appetizer.

TIP: You can make your own roasted red peppers using the following technique: Preheat the oven to 450°F. Rinse and dry red bell peppers and place on a small baking sheet. Roast until the skins are charred, 25 to 30 minutes, rotating at the halfway point. Remove the peppers from the oven and place in a bowl to cool. Once cooled, gently remove the stem, then peel off the skin and remove the inner membrane and seeds.

PER SERVING: Calories: 192; Total fat: 4 g; Saturated fat: 1 g; Cholesterol: 1 mg; Sodium: 73 mg; Potassium: 411 mg; Total carbohydrates: 29 g; Fiber: 8 g; Sugars: 7 g; Protein: 11 g

Coconut Rice and White Beans

This flavorful dish is a fusion of several cuisines, including those found in the Caribbean and Asia, and is simple to prep for busy weeknights. In this version of rice and beans, black rice (also marketed as Forbidden Rice) is used to boost the antioxidant content, and is combined with healthy high-protein white beans, which are simmered in light coconut milk to create a lovely creamy texture while keeping fat in check. Lemongrass gives it a strong citrus fragrance and taste and it has plenty of Caribbean-inspired spices as well, including garlic, cinnamon, and lime. Vegan and gluten-free, this filling and comforting dish is packed full of interesting tastes.

1 stalk lemongrass, bottom 6 inches only, outer leaves peeled

1 teaspoon extra-virgin olive oil

2 cloves garlic, minced

2 tablespoons minced shallot

½ cup chopped red bell pepper

1 cup cubed and peeled eggplant

1 teaspoon ground cardamom

1 teaspoon ground coriander

½ teaspoon ground cinnamon

½ cup canned no-salt-added diced tomatoes and their juices

½ cup black rice (see Tip)

⅔ cup canned "lite" coconut milk

1 (15-ounce) can small white beans, rinsed and drained

2 cups chopped baby kale

½ lime

Hot sauce (optional)

Salt and freshly ground black pepper (optional)

1. Lightly pound the lemongrass stalk with a kitchen mallet.

2. In a large pot, heat the olive oil over high heat. Add the garlic and shallot and cook until soft, 3 to 5 minutes. Add the bell pepper and eggplant and continue cooking until softened, 3 to 5 minutes.

3. Add the cardamom, coriander, and cinnamon and cook for 1 more minute, stirring occasionally to prevent the spices from burning.

4. Add the tomatoes, black rice, coconut milk, 1½ cups water, and beans and stir to combine. Cover, bring to a boil, then reduce the heat to low and allow to simmer for 20 minutes.

5. Stir in the kale, cover, and continue cooking until the kale is wilted, the rice is done, and most of the liquid is absorbed, 5 to 8 minutes longer.

6. To serve, remove the lemongrass stalk and squeeze in the lime juice. If desired, season with hot sauce and a dash of salt and black pepper.

TIP: Black rice can be found in most major grocery stores with the other types of rice. It's higher in antioxidants than other rice, creates a striking dish, and kids love the different look! If you can't find it, substitute another whole-grain rice, but be certain to adjust the cooking time according to the package directions.

PER SERVING: Calories: 433; Total fat: 9 g; Saturated fat: 5 g; Cholesterol: 0 mg; Sodium: 32 mg; Potassium: 474 mg; Total carbohydrates: 75 g; Fiber: 16 g; Sugars: 6 g; Protein: 19 g

Creamy Cauliflower Butternut Squash Mac and Cheese

You can still enjoy the classic comfort food, macaroni and cheese, while watching your weight and keeping your blood pressure in check by sneaking in some additional veggies and combining low-fat, high-protein ricotta cheese with cheddar cheese. The perfect compromise to a normally carb- and fat-laden dish, this version also uses chickpea pasta to boost the protein and fiber content. The result is a filling, healthy meal with all of the creamy deliciousness of the original but far less sodium, fat, and refined carbohydrates.

8 ounces chickpea pasta elbows (see Tips, page 135)

2 cups cubed peeled butternut squash

2 cups cauliflower florets

2 cups fat-free milk

½ teaspoon freshly ground black pepper

Dash of salt

½ tablespoon extra-virgin olive oil

½ medium red onion, minced

2 cloves garlic, minced

2 teaspoons Dijon mustard

2 teaspoons sweet paprika

1 cup shredded low-fat cheddar cheese

½ cup part-skim ricotta cheese

TIP: One cup of cooked butternut squash has more potassium than a banana, provides over 160% of your daily recommended intake of vitamin A, and contains a healthy dose of B vitamins (including folate), vitamin C, and dietary fiber.

1. Cook the pasta according to the package directions. Drain and set aside.

2. In a medium saucepan, combine the butternut squash, cauliflower, and 1 cup of the milk. Season with the pepper and salt. Bring to a simmer over medium-high heat, then reduce the heat to low, cover, and cook until fork-tender, 8 to 10 minutes. Transfer the cooked vegetables to a food processor or blender and puree until smooth.

3. Meanwhile, in a large saucepan, heat the olive oil over medium-high heat. Add the onion and garlic and sauté until tender, 3 to 5 minutes.

4. Add the vegetable puree, the remaining 1 cup milk, the mustard, and paprika to the saucepan and bring to a simmer. Cook until starting to thicken, about 5 minutes.

5. Add the cheddar and ricotta cheese and stir to combine. Add the drained pasta to the pan and stir to combine.

6. Serve immediately.

PER SERVING: Calories: 372; Total fat: 9 g; Saturated fat: 2 g; Cholesterol: 15 mg; Sodium: 405 mg; Potassium: 616 mg; Total carbohydrates: 53 g; Fiber: 13 g; Sugars: 13 g; Protein: 28 g

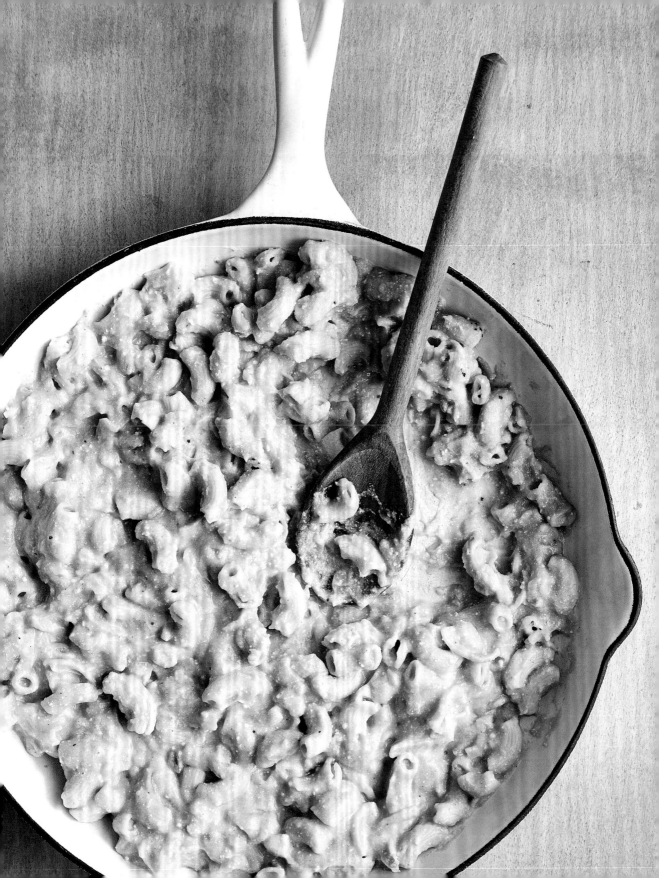

Two-Pea Jollof Rice

When I was in the Peace Corps in Sierra Leone, West Africa, jollof rice was one of my favorite dishes. Said to have originated from the Wolof tribe in Senegal, every country and tribe has its own version, and each abhors the others' "inauthentic" variations. While my version would probably fall into the latter category, it does maintain some of the distinctive flavors through the use of onion, chili peppers, tomatoes, tomato paste, and signature spices including cumin and ginger. This vegan version doesn't contain any "bush meat" or use red palm oil, but it is most delicious, protein and fiber rich, and certain to satisfy.

- 2 teaspoons extra-virgin olive oil
- ½ cup chopped onion
- 2 cloves garlic, minced
- 1 teaspoon minced peeled fresh ginger
- 2 fresh Thai chili peppers or Scotch bonnet peppers (see Tip), sliced
- ¼ teaspoon salt
- ½ cup brown basmati rice
- 1 teaspoon ground coriander
- 1 teaspoon dried thyme
- ½ teaspoon ground cumin
- ½ teaspoon sweet paprika
- 1 cup canned no-salt-added diced tomatoes with their juices
- 2 tablespoons tomato paste
- 1 cup low-sodium vegetable broth
- ⅔ cup frozen green peas
- 1 cup canned black-eyed peas, drained and rinsed
- ¼ cup chopped fresh parsley (optional)

1. In a large soup pot or Dutch oven, heat the olive oil over medium-high heat. Add the onion and cook, stirring frequently, until starting to turn translucent, 4 to 5 minutes. Mix in the garlic, ginger, and chili peppers and cook for 30 seconds, until the spices turn fragrant. Add the salt and basmati rice and stir. Continue toasting the rice for 2 minutes.

2. Add the coriander, thyme, cumin, paprika, diced tomatoes, tomato paste, vegetable broth, green peas, and black-eyed peas and stir until well combined. Cover, reduce the heat to medium-low, and simmer until all of the liquid is absorbed and the stew has thickened, 35 to 40 minutes. Don't lift the lid during cooking.

3. Remove the pan from the heat and let sit for 8 to 10 minutes to let the rice finish cooking.

4. Fluff with a fork and serve immediately, sprinkled with fresh parsley, if desired.

TIP: If you can't find fresh Thai chili peppers or Scotch bonnet peppers, you can substitute dried. These can usually be found in the spice section packaged in small bags. Alternatively, use cayenne pepper or red pepper flakes.

PER SERVING: Calories: 407; Total fat: 6 g; Saturated fat: <1 g; Cholesterol: 0 mg; Sodium: 536 mg; Potassium: 586 mg; Total carbohydrates: 74 g; Fiber: 14 g; Sugars: 11 g; Protein: 15 g

Bean Pasta with Arugula Avocado Walnut Pesto

You don't have to give up on pasta or pesto when following the DASH diet for weight loss. Instead, you just have to make a few smart substitutions to keep the flavor and satisfaction level high while reducing sodium, unhealthy fats, and excess calories. Store-bought pesto is typically very high in sodium, fat, and calories for a teeny, tiny serving size. But this recipe makes plenty to coat protein-rich bean pasta with enough creamy goodness to keep you feeling satisfied. Quick to prepare, this is a hearty, flavorful plant-based meal that is also gluten-free and vegan.

2 cups packed arugula

1 cup packed fresh basil leaves

¼ cup chopped walnuts

⅔ cup green peas (thawed if frozen)

½ medium avocado

3 cloves garlic, coarsely chopped

2 tablespoons fresh lemon juice

¼ cup nutritional yeast (see Tips)

Pinch of salt

3 tablespoons extra-virgin olive oil

8 ounces bean pasta (see Tips)

Fresh parsley (optional)

1. Fill a large saucepan three-quarters full with water and bring to a rolling boil over high heat.

2. Meanwhile, in a food processor, combine the arugula, basil, walnuts, peas, avocado, garlic, lemon juice, nutritional yeast, and salt and pulse until finely chopped. Add the olive oil and continue to process the pesto until creamy or the desired consistency is reached.

3. Add the pasta to the boiling water and cook to al dente, according to the package directions, being certain not to overcook. Drain the pasta and transfer to a bowl. Add the pesto and toss to combine.

4. Portion onto 4 serving plates and garnish with fresh parsley, if desired.

TIPS: You can omit the nutritional yeast or substitute an equal amount of freshly grated Parmesan if you are not vegan. Just note that this change will affect the nutritional analysis.

Bean pasta is a dream come true for health-conscious individuals looking to manage their weight while boosting their nutrition. Readily available in grocery stores, Banza is a brand of chickpea pasta that has gone mainstream. Incredibly satisfying with a creamy beanlike consistency but in pasta form, a single serving has double the protein and fiber of traditional pasta.

PER SERVING: Calories: 417; Total fat: 22 g; Saturated fat: 2 g; Cholesterol: 0 mg; Sodium: 122 mg; Potassium: 289 mg; Total carbohydrates: 43 g; Fiber: 13 g; Sugars: 7 g; Protein: 21 g

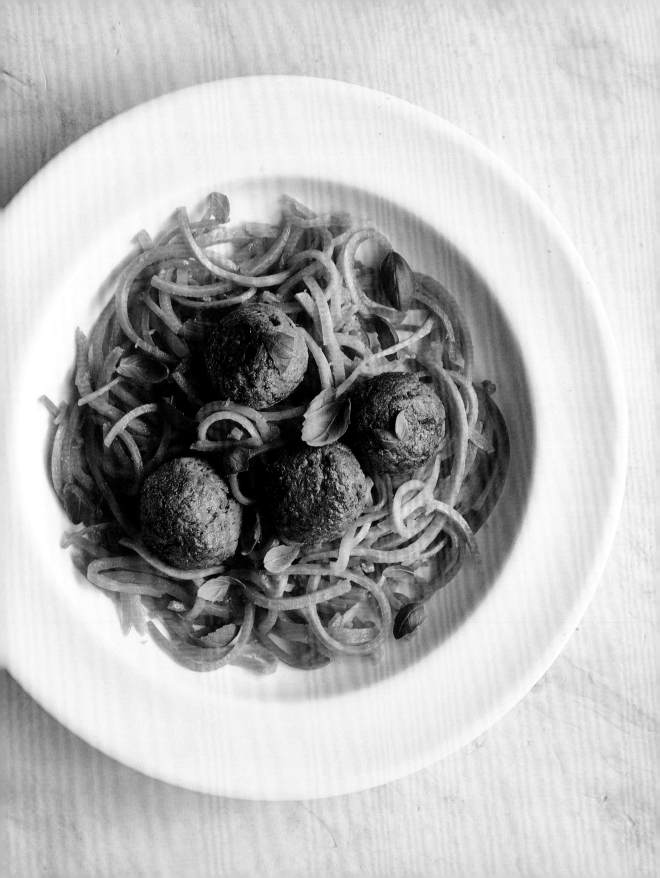

PREP TIME: 30 MINUTES • COOK TIME: 30 MINUTES • SERVES 4

Tofu, Carrot, and Walnut "Meatballs" over Butternut Squash Noodles

These delicious "meatballs" made using tofu, vegetables, and walnuts are a great meat-free alternative, and are delicious served over vegetable noodles. Rich tasting with a hint of sweetness, the nutritional yeast adds a bit of vegan "cheese" flavor.

1 (14-ounce) block firm tofu

1½ tablespoons extra-virgin olive oil

4 cloves garlic, minced

1 cup coarsely chopped red onion

1 cup grated carrot

½ cup walnuts, chopped

¼ cup frozen shelled edamame

1 tablespoon Bragg liquid aminos

2 teaspoons dried oregano

1½ teaspoons fennel seeds

1 teaspoon red pepper flakes

¼ cup coconut flour

3 tablespoons nutritional yeast

1 to 2 tablespoons fresh lemon juice

1 (10-ounce) package butternut squash noodles

½ cup chopped fresh basil leaves

Salt and freshly ground black pepper (optional)

1. Use a tofu press or pat the tofu dry and roll in a clean absorbent towel and place something heavy on top such as a heavy skillet or plates with a can on top, for at least 15 minutes (up to 1 hour) in order to remove excess water.

2. Preheat the oven to 350°F. Coat a large baking sheet with cooking spray or line with parchment paper.

3. In a medium skillet, heat 1 tablespoon of the olive oil over medium-high heat. Add the garlic, onion, and carrot and sauté until soft, 3 to 5 minutes. Remove from the heat and set aside.

4. In a food processor, pulse the walnuts until they are coarsely ground.

5. To the food processor, add the tofu, edamame, Bragg aminos, oregano, fennel seeds, pepper flakes, coconut flour, nutritional yeast, and sautéed vegetables and blend slowly until combined, adding the lemon juice 1 tablespoon at a time until the mixture is moist enough to hold together.

6. Form the mixture into 12 balls (a little bigger than a golf ball) and place on the prepared baking sheet. Bake for 15 minutes, then flip over and continue baking until lightly browned, about 15 minutes more.

7. During the last 10 minutes of baking, heat the remaining ½ tablespoon olive oil in the skillet over medium-high heat. Add the butternut squash noodles and lightly sauté until warmed through, 3 to 5 minutes.

8. Divide the squash noodles among 4 serving plates, top each plate with 3 meatballs, garnish with fresh basil, and season with salt and pepper, if desired.

PER SERVING: Calories: 369; Total fat: 22 g; Saturated fat: 2 g; Cholesterol: 0 mg; Sodium: 520 mg; Potassium: 527 mg; Total carbohydrates: 31 g; Fiber: 10 g; Sugars: 5 g; Protein: 21 g

Lentil Sloppy Joes

A plant-based version of a classic comfort food and summertime favorite, these tasty lentil sloppy Joes contain a hearty mix of vegetables and spices that pack as much flavor and protein as the original, but with far more fiber, vitamins, and minerals, and no unhealthy fats. Slightly spicy and naturally sweetened with dried apricots, these sloppy Joes are both kid friendly and freezer friendly. Serve on top of lettuce leaves or on whole-grain buns with your favorite fixings.

1 cup green or brown lentils, rinsed

¼ cup unsweetened dried apricots, chopped

2 tablespoons tomato paste

½ teaspoon yellow mustard

½ tablespoon extra-virgin olive oil

½ medium yellow onion, diced

1 medium green bell pepper, diced

1 large stalk celery, diced

½ cup grated carrot

3 cloves garlic, minced

1 (15-ounce) can tomato sauce

1 tablespoon red wine vinegar

1 tablespoon vegetarian Worcestershire sauce (see Tip)

2 teaspoons chili powder

1 teaspoon ground cumin

1 teaspoon smoked or sweet paprika

Lettuce leaves or whole-grain buns

TIP: Worcestershire sauce contains anchovies, so to keep this vegan/vegetarian, choose a vegetarian version. This should be easy to find right alongside regular Worcestershire sauce in the grocery store.

1. In a small saucepan, combine the lentils and 2 cups water. Bring to a boil, reduce the heat, and simmer, covered, until tender but not falling apart, 20 to 25 minutes. Drain and set aside.

2. Meanwhile, in a food processor or blender, combine the dried apricots, tomato paste, and mustard and process/blend until the apricots are blended into a paste. Transfer the apricot paste to a small bowl and set aside.

3. Heat a large skillet over medium-high heat. Add the olive oil, onion, bell pepper, celery, carrot, and garlic and stir to combine. Cook, stirring frequently, until the vegetables are slightly browned and tender, 4 to 5 minutes.

4. Add the apricot paste, tomato sauce, vinegar, Worcestershire sauce, chili powder, cumin, and paprika to the skillet. Stir to combine and cook until the spices are fragrant, 2 minutes.

5. Add the drained lentils to the pan and stir well to combine. Continue cooking over medium-low heat until the sauce thickens, stirring occasionally, 5 to 10 minutes. Taste and adjust seasonings before serving.

6. Ladle the mixture onto lettuce leaves or toasted buns.

PER SERVING (WITHOUT BUN): Calories: 269; Total fat: 3 g; Saturated fat: <1 g; Cholesterol: 0 mg; Sodium: 559 mg; Potassium: 804 mg; Total carbohydrates: 50 g; Fiber: 17 g; Sugars: 13 g; Protein: 15 g

Lentil-Walnut Mushroom Tacos

Cooked lentils, smoky chipotle peppers, and meaty pistachios, walnuts, and mushrooms are combined and baked into a crumbly mixture. The lentil-nut "taco meat" is then used to stuff hearty, rich portobello mushrooms to create a filling and satisfying meal rich in nutrients yet surprisingly low in calories.

¼ cup green or brown lentils, rinsed

4 portobello mushrooms

¼ cup unsalted pistachios

¼ cup walnut halves

2 tablespoons chopped canned chipotle peppers in adobo sauce

2 cups riced cauliflower

1 teaspoon chili powder

1 teaspoon ground coriander

1 teaspoon ground cumin

1 teaspoon garlic powder

1 teaspoon dried oregano

1 teaspoon smoked paprika

Juice of 1 lime

1. In a small saucepan, cook the lentils in water to cover over medium-high heat until tender, 20 to 25 minutes. Drain and set aside.

2. Meanwhile, preheat the oven to 375°F. Line a large baking sheet with parchment paper.

3. Remove the stems and carefully scrape out the gills from the mushrooms using a small paring knife. Transfer to a food processor.

4. In a dry medium skillet, toast the pistachios and walnuts, stirring constantly, until lightly golden, 2 to 3 minutes.

5. Scrape the nuts into the food processor. Add the chipotle peppers in adobo sauce and the drained lentils. Pulse lightly until the ingredients are combined, being careful not to overprocess as you want there to be some texture.

6. In a medium bowl, combine the riced cauliflower, chili powder, coriander cumin, garlic powder, oregano, and paprika. Add the contents of the food processor to the bowl and mix until everything is combined.

7. Spread the mixture on the parchment and drizzle with lime juice. Bake for 15 minutes. Use a spatula to turn the mixture, and also make room for the portobello mushroom caps. Coat both sides of the caps lightly with cooking spray. Return to the oven and bake until the mushroom caps are lightly browned and the lentil mixture is lightly browned and crumbly but not overly dry, 15 minutes to 20 minutes longer.

8. Remove the pan from the oven and give the lentil mixture a good stir.

9. To serve, place 2 mushroom caps on each of 2 serving plates and top with the lentil-nut "meat."

PER SERVING: Calories: 346; Total fat: 19 g; Saturated fat: 2 g; Cholesterol: 0 mg; Sodium: 141 mg; Potassium: 1,212 mg; Total carbohydrates: 33 g; Fiber: 15 g; Sugars: 16 g; Protein: 19 g

The Best Black Bean and Beet Burger

Homemade veggie burgers are a cinch to make, and so much healthier than processed varieties. Black beans, rolled oats, and beets are combined with herbs and spices and a bit of flour to create a super-satisfying veggie burger packed with blood-pressure-lowering nutrients that holds together beautifully. A bonus is that you won't even know the beets are there, so this is also a great choice for boosting the veggie intake of little ones in the house. Serve open-faced on lettuce leaves or on a whole-grain bun with your favorite sides.

1 tablespoon chia seeds

1 (15-ounce) can black beans, rinsed and drained

¼ pound cooked and peeled beets, quartered (2 medium)

½ cup steel-cut oats

1 cup sliced mushrooms

1 teaspoon dry mustard

1 teaspoon ground cumin

½ teaspoon smoked paprika

1 teaspoon Bragg liquid aminos or reduced-sodium soy sauce

1 teaspoon vegan Worcestershire sauce

1 teaspoon minced garlic

Pinch of salt

2 tablespoons chickpea flour (see Tips) or other whole-grain flour, plus more as needed

Lettuce leaves or whole-grain buns

1. In a small bowl, combine the chia seeds and 3 tablespoons water to make a chia "egg." Set aside for 5 minutes, until the mixture forms a gel.

2. Meanwhile, in a medium bowl, coarsely mash ½ cup of the black beans with a fork, leaving some texture.

3. In a food processor, combine the remaining black beans, the chia "egg," beets, oats, mushrooms, mustard, cumin, paprika, liquid aminos, Worcestershire sauce, garlic, and salt. Pulse until the ingredients are combined but not completely pulverized. You want the burgers to have some texture.

4. Add the contents of the food processor to the bowl with the mashed beans. Add the chickpea flour and mix (it might be easier to use your hands) until the ingredients hold together, adding more flour as needed. Refrigerate to chill for 10 minutes while you preheat the oven. Chilling helps the burgers hold together better.

5. Preheat the oven to 375°F. Coat a baking sheet with cooking spray.

6. Remove the mixture from the fridge and form it into 6 evenly sized balls, then use the palm of your hand to gently flatten into patties.

7. Arrange the burgers on the baking sheet and lightly spray the tops with cooking spray. Bake for 30 minutes to heat through, until lightly browned, gently turning halfway through cooking.

8. Serve on lettuce leaves or toasted whole-grain buns.

PER SERVING (WITHOUT BUN): Calories: 132; Total fat: 1 g; Saturated fat: <1 g; Cholesterol: 0 mg; Sodium: 89 mg; Potassium: 103 mg; Total carbohydrates: 24 g; Fiber: 6 g; Sugars: 2 g; Protein: 7 g

TIPS: These burgers freeze really well. To do this, partially bake them at 375°F for 15 to 20 minutes, until they firm up. Allow the burgers to cool, then wrap in parchment and place in a freezer bag and freeze for up to 1 month. To cook, place on a baking sheet and bake at 375°F for 25 to 30 minutes, until desired doneness.

You can swap in almond meal/flour for the chickpea flour for a slightly different taste and texture. Just note that doing this will change the nutritional content and add slightly more calories and fat.

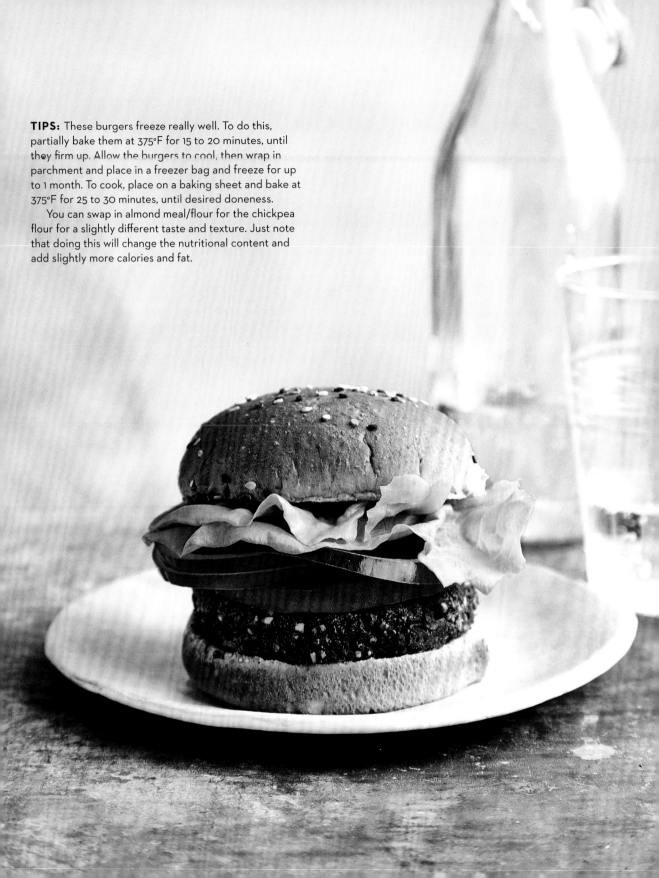

PREP TIME: 10 MINUTES · COOK TIME: 15 MINUTES · SERVES 4

Cauliflower "Fried Rice" and Mixed Vegetables

Riced cauliflower is a true waistline and heart health saver for fans of Chinese fried rice. So much healthier than refined carbohydrate- and unhealthy fat-laden traditional fried rice, this nutritious version is packed with fiber-rich vegetables and protein. To keep sodium in check, the vegetables are cooked in flavorful sesame oil with a touch of balsamic vinegar and soy sauce, which complements the earthy taste of the cauliflower. Cook this like you would any stir-fry using a very hot skillet or wok while stirring quickly. Super delicious and quick to prepare, mix up the vegetables based on your personal preferences.

1 tablespoon + 1 teaspoon sesame oil

1 cup chopped scallions, white and green parts separated

2 cloves garlic, minced

1 teaspoon grated fresh ginger

1 red bell pepper, chopped

1 cup frozen shelled edamame, thawed

1 cup mushrooms, sliced

4 cups fresh or frozen riced cauliflower (see Tip)

2 egg whites, whisked

1 large egg, beaten

1 tablespoon reduced-sodium soy sauce

1 tablespoon balsamic vinegar

Pinch of red pepper flakes

¼ cup chopped peanuts or cashews

1. In a large wok or nonstick skillet, heat 1 tablespoon of the sesame oil over medium-high heat. Add the scallion whites, garlic, and ginger and cook, stirring often, until fragrant but not browned, 2 to 3 minutes.

2. Add the bell pepper, edamame, and mushrooms and cook until the pepper is softened, about 2 minutes. Add the cauliflower rice, stir to combine, and stir-fry quickly to cook the cauliflower to a soft but not mushy texture, 5 to 7 minutes.

3. Make a well in the center of the vegetables. Reduce the heat, add the remaining 1 teaspoon sesame oil to the center, and add the egg whites and whole egg. Stir gently and constantly until the eggs are fully cooked, then stir together with the cauliflower rice.

4. Stir in the scallion greens, the soy sauce, balsamic vinegar, and pepper flakes and cook for 1 minute.

5. Serve garnished with chopped nuts.

TIP: While riced cauliflower is readily available, a time saver, and budget friendly, you can certainly start with a head of cauliflower and rice it using a food processor. Simply cut the florets from the stem into 1-inch pieces. Add them to a food processor and pulse until small pieces form, scraping the sides of the bowl as needed.

PER SERVING: Calories: 219; Total fat: 12 g; Saturated fat: 2 g; Cholesterol: 46 mg; Sodium: 219 mg; Potassium: 497 mg; Total carbohydrates: 17 g; Fiber: 6 g; Sugars: 4 g; Protein: 15 g

Crustless Vegan Mushroom and Sweet Potato Mini Quiches

This is one of my go-to recipes that I make just about every week and never get tired of. It's super fast to prep and you can create endless variations depending on what you are in the mood for. Make two large ones as a main course, or four smaller ones to use as healthy snacks or sides. These are extremely filling and satisfying, full of protein, fiber, and essential vitamins and minerals, so even if you aren't vegan, please give this recipe a try!

1 cup chickpea flour

¼ cup nutritional yeast

1 teaspoon baking powder

2 teaspoons ground sage

1 teaspoon dried thyme

1 teaspoon ground turmeric

Pinch of salt (black salt, if possible; see Tip)

Freshly ground black pepper

1 cup unsweetened cashew milk (or fat-free dairy milk if you are not vegan)

⅔ cup frozen green peas, slightly thawed

1 cup riced cauliflower and sweet potato (see Tip)

1 cup finely chopped button mushrooms

1 teaspoon minced garlic

1 tablespoon minced shallot

1. Preheat the oven to 375°F. For a main course, lightly coat four 1-cup ramekins with cooking spray; for a snack or side, spray 8 cups of a muffin tin.

2. In a medium bowl, stir together the chickpea flour, nutritional yeast, baking powder, sage, thyme, turmeric, salt, and black pepper to taste. Stir in the milk.

3. Add the peas, riced cauliflower and sweet potato, mushrooms, garlic, and shallot and mix to combine. The batter will be thin.

4. Divide the batter evenly among the prepared ramekins or muffin cups. Transfer to the oven and bake until firm to the touch and lightly browned, about 35 minutes.

5. Remove from the oven and let sit for an additional 10 minutes (they will continue to firm up), then transfer to a wire rack and allow to cool slightly if eating immediately or completely if storing for later. Store in an airtight container in the refrigerator for up to 1 week.

TIP: Black salt is used in a lot of vegan recipes. It has a sulfur smell and taste and adds an egg-like flavor. You only need a very small amount, as the taste is very strong. You can find it online.

PER MAIN-COURSE SERVING: Calories: 356; Total fat: 1 g; Saturated fat: <1 g; Cholesterol: 0 mg; Sodium: 178 mg; Potassium: 506 mg; Total carbohydrates: 57 g; Fiber: 16 g; Sugars: 11 g; Protein: 23 g

PER SNACK/SIDE SERVING: Calories: 178; Total fat: <1 g; Saturated fat: <1 g; Cholesterol: 0 mg; Sodium: 89 mg; Potassium: 253 mg; Total carbohydrates: 29 g; Fiber: 8 g; Sugars: 5 g; Protein: 12 g

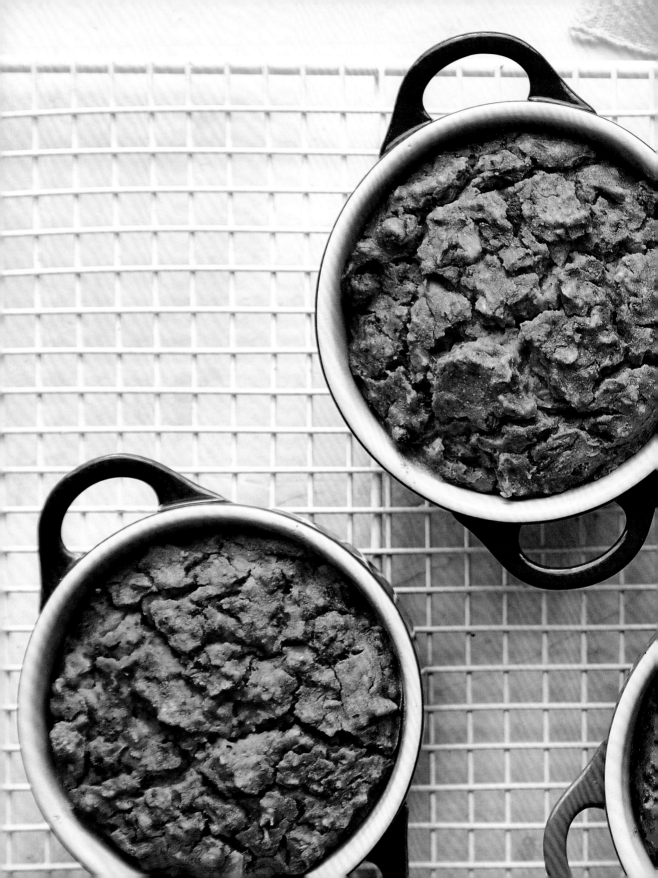

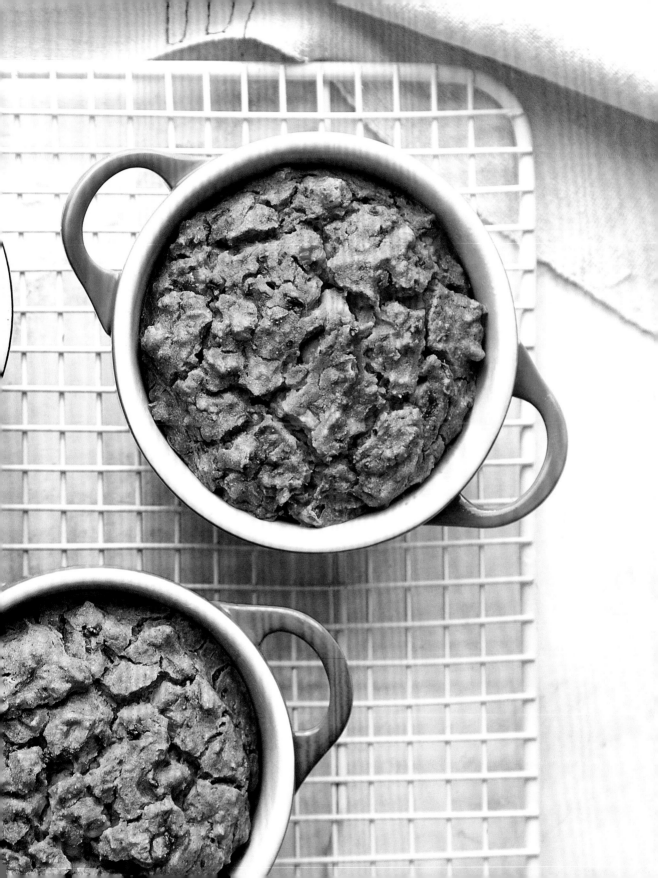

Tofu Scramble with Broccoli and Sun-Dried Tomatoes

Tofu scramble is a classic vegan recipe with endless variations that is simple to master and a great addition to your "go-to" list of quick and easy meal ideas. Don't let tofu intimidate you, or the fear of the unknown put you off preparing it.

1 (14-ounce) block extra-firm tofu

SAUCE

1 teaspoon ground cumin

1 teaspoon ground turmeric

½ teaspoon chili powder

½ teaspoon freshly ground black pepper

½ tablespoon reduced-sodium soy sauce or Bragg liquid aminos

SCRAMBLE

1 tablespoon extra-virgin olive oil

1 red bell pepper, thinly sliced

½ medium onion, thinly sliced

2 cloves garlic, minced

1 cup broccoli florets

1 (15-ounce) can black beans, rinsed and drained

¼ cup julienned dry-packed sun-dried tomatoes

OPTIONAL TOPPINGS

Avocado slices

Chopped fresh cilantro

Hot sauce

1. Pat the tofu dry and roll it in a clean absorbent towel; place something heavy on top such as a skillet or plates with a can on top for at least 15 minutes (up to 1 hour) in order to remove excess water.

2. While the tofu is draining, prepare the sauce: In a small bowl, whisk together the cumin, turmeric, chili powder, black pepper, and soy sauce. The sauce should have some body and not be too runny.

3. Make the scramble: In a large skillet, heat the olive oil over medium heat. Add the bell pepper and onion and cook until softened, about 5 minutes. Add the garlic and cook for 1 minute.

4. Add the broccoli; cover and steam for 2 minutes.

5. Meanwhile, unwrap the tofu and use a fork to crumble into bite-size pieces.

6. Use a spatula and move the vegetables to one side of the skillet. Add the crumbled tofu and sauté for 2 to 3 minutes, until lightly browned, then combine with the vegetables, pour in the sauce, and cook for another 3 minutes, until the tofu is evenly coated and has absorbed some of the sauce.

7. Add the beans and sun-dried tomatoes and continue cooking until the tofu is lightly browned, another 5 to 7 minutes.

8. Serve with the optional toppings, if desired.

PER SERVING: Calories: 251; Total fat: 8 g; Saturated fat: 1 g; Cholesterol: 0 mg; Sodium: 98 mg; Potassium: 358 mg; Total carbohydrates: 28 g; Fiber: 7 g; Sugars: 3 g; Protein: 18 g

Almond Butter Tofu and Roasted Asparagus

This rich-tasting and flavorful tofu stir-fry is made using an almond butter–based marinade for the tofu, which is baked and then lightly browned in a skillet and served with juicy roasted asparagus. Full of plant-powered protein, healthy fats, blood-pressure-lowering nutrients, and gut-friendly prebiotics, this simple dish will satisfy your cravings for Asian food without excess calories and unhealthy fats. Serve as is or over brown rice or Herbed Cauliflower and Broccoli Rice (page 211).

1 (14-ounce) block extra-firm tofu

1 tablespoon sesame oil

1 tablespoon pure maple syrup

2 tablespoons reduced-sodium tamari

2 tablespoons almond butter

2 tablespoons fresh lime juice

1 tablespoon balsamic vinegar

3 cloves garlic, minced

1 pound asparagus, tough ends trimmed

1 tablespoon extra-virgin olive oil

Freshly ground black pepper (optional)

Chili hot sauce (e.g. Sriracha) (optional)

1. Pat tofu dry and roll in a clean absorbent towel and place something heavy on top such as a heavy skillet or plates with a can on top, for at least 15 minutes (up to 1 hour) in order to remove excess water.

2. Preheat the oven to 400°F. Coat two large baking sheets with cooking spray.

3. Unwrap the tofu and cut into 1-inch cubes. Arrange on one of the prepared baking sheets in an even layer and bake until puffy and slightly browned, 20 to 25 minutes.

4. Meanwhile, in a small bowl, combine the sesame oil, maple syrup, tamari, almond butter, lime juice, balsamic vinegar, and two-thirds of the minced garlic. Whisk to combine. Set the marinade aside.

5. In a medium bowl, drizzle the asparagus with the olive oil, then toss to coat. Sprinkle with the remaining garlic and season with black pepper, if desired. Arrange the asparagus in a single layer on the second baking sheet.

6. Remove the tofu from the oven and place the asparagus in the oven in its place. Add the baked tofu to the marinade and toss to coat. Let marinate for 5 minutes, stirring occasionally.

7. Heat a large skillet over medium heat. Once hot, add the tofu (reserve the marinade) and cook, stirring occasionally, until browned on all sides, about 5 minutes.

8. Remove the roasted asparagus from the oven and add to the skillet with the tofu along with the reserved marinade. Cook for an additional 2 minutes, stirring frequently.

9. Garnish with hot sauce, if desired.

TIP: Balsamic vinegar replaces part of the tamari that would normally be used in this type of recipe, a technique you can use when preparing stir-fry recipes to maintain the distinctive flavor that tamari and soy sauce impart while keeping sodium in check.

PER SERVING: Calories: 337; Total fat: 21 g; Saturated fat: 3 g; Cholesterol: 0 mg; Sodium: 496 mg; Potassium: 528 mg; Total carbohydrates: 21 g; Fiber: 6 g; Sugars: 8 g; Protein: 21 g

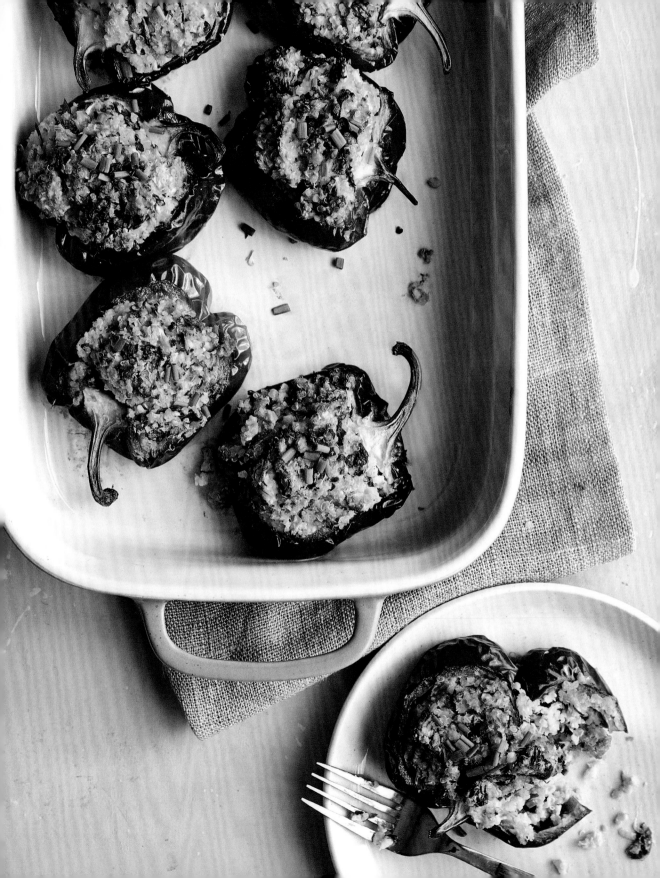

Quinoa and Red Lentil Stuffed Peppers with a Creamy Cashew Sauce

If you are transitioning to a more plant based diet and are looking for dishes that are as satisfying as those made with meat, then I highly recommend you try this recipe. Super flavorful, hearty, filling, and delicious, this protein and fiber-packed vegan recipe is quick to prepare, and a healthy meal the entire family will love.

½ cup quinoa, rinsed

½ cup red lentils (see Tip), rinsed

½ cup raw cashews

¼ cup fresh lemon juice

3 to 4 teaspoons minced garlic

1 cup fresh basil leaves

Pinch of salt

¼ teaspoon freshly ground black pepper

1 cup riced cauliflower (see Tip, page 142)

2 cups baby spinach or baby kale, chopped

¼ cup nutritional yeast

2 teaspoons dried thyme

Pinch of cayenne pepper

4 large bell peppers, any color, halved lengthwise

Fresh chives (optional)

1. In a saucepan, combine the quinoa, lentils, and 2 cups water and bring to a boil over high heat. Reduce the heat, cover, and simmer until the liquid is absorbed, the quinoa is fluffy, and the lentils are tender, 15 to 20 minutes.

2. Preheat the oven to 375°F. Pour ½ inch water into a baking dish big enough to hold the pepper halves in a single layer.

3. Meanwhile, in a food processor or high-powered blender, combine the cashews, ½ cup water, the lemon juice, garlic to taste, basil, salt, and black pepper and process until creamy and smooth. Pour into a medium bowl.

4. To the bowl, add the cooked quinoa and lentils, riced cauliflower, spinach, nutritional yeast, thyme, and cayenne. Mix thoroughly to combine.

5. Lightly spray the halved peppers with nonstick cooking spray and place cut side up in the baking dish. Dividing evenly, spoon the filling into each bell pepper cavity until full. Cover with foil and bake for 30 minutes. Remove the foil and bake until the peppers are soft and slightly golden brown, another 15 to 20 minutes.

6. Garnish with fresh chives, if desired, and serve immediately.

TIP: Red lentils are used in this recipe because they have a shorter cooking time and break down or disintegrate when cooked, which adds to the creamy texture of this recipe. They are also sweeter than brown or green lentils and add a nice bright color to the dish. Or you can add your favorite canned bean (cannellini, for example) instead of lentils: Simply omit the lentils and cook the quinoa in 1 cup water following the same cooking directions as above. Then add 1 cup beans to the bowl of ingredients in step 4.

PER SERVING: Calories: 326; Total fat: 9 g; Saturated fat: 0 g; Cholesterol: 0 mg; Sodium: 73 mg; Potassium: 575 mg; Total carbohydrates: 47 g; Fiber: 14 g; Sugars: 8 g; Protein: 17 g

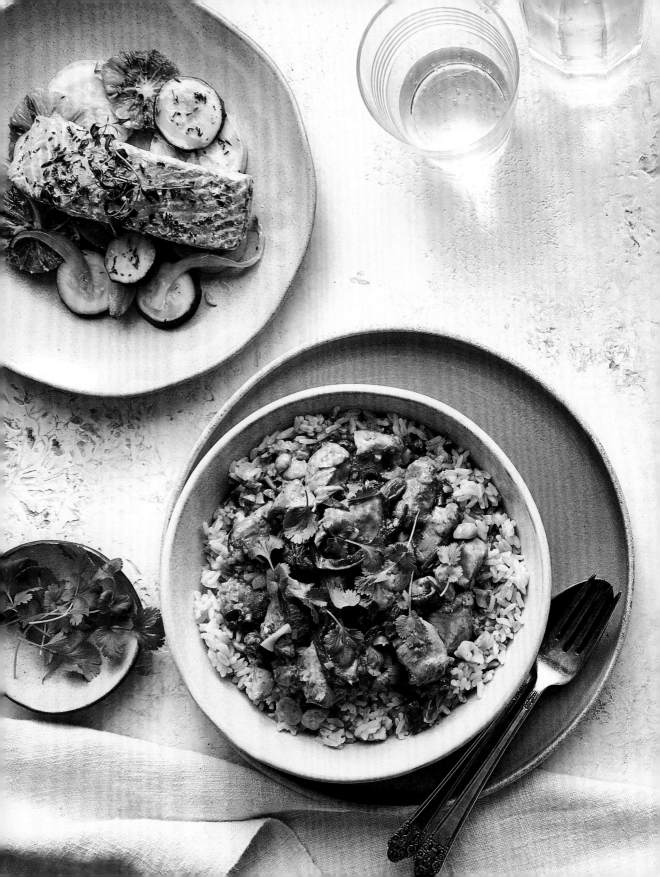

Poultry and Fish

Chicken and Vegetable Stir-Fry

Stir-fry dishes are a great option on busy nights as the prep and cooking time are minimal if you buy prechopped vegetables, and you can improvise with whatever vegetables you have on hand. Stir-frying is usually done in a wok as its high sides increase the cooking surface you have, but if you don't have one, you can use a large sauté pan. Low in sodium yet full of flavor, serve as is or over riced cauliflower or brown rice.

2 tablespoons sesame oil

1 pound boneless, skinless chicken breasts, cubed

3 cloves garlic, minced

½ of an 8-ounce package sugar snap peas

4 scallions, chopped

1 (16-ounce) bag frozen stir-fry vegetables, thawed

8 ounces water chestnuts, drained and rinsed

2 teaspoons Chinese five-spice powder

2 teaspoons reduced-sodium soy sauce

2 tablespoons balsamic vinegar

2 teaspoons hot sauce

1. In a wok or large sauté pan, heat ½ tablespoon of the sesame oil over medium heat. Add the chicken and cook until lightly browned, 5 to 7 minutes. Transfer the chicken to a bowl, cover, and set aside.

2. Add the remaining 1½ tablespoons sesame oil to the pan along with the garlic and snap peas. Cook until the peas begin to soften and the garlic begins to brown, 3 to 4 minutes. Add the scallions, stir-fry vegetables, and water chestnuts and cook, stirring constantly, for 2 minutes.

3. Add the five-spice powder, soy sauce, balsamic vinegar, and hot sauce. Return the cooked chicken to the pan and stir, cooking for 2 additional minutes, until the chicken is warmed through and the ingredients are combined.

TIPS: Five-spice powder is a blend of cinnamon, cloves, fennel, star anise, and Sichuan peppercorns.

Even reduced-sodium soy sauce has over 500 milligrams of sodium in 1 tablespoon. A good trick to keep the distinctive flavor while keeping sodium in check is to use just a small amount of soy sauce and make up the flavor with vinegar and spices. Balsamic goes well with chicken, red wine vinegar goes well with beef, and rice vinegar goes well with vegetables. Hot sauce adds heat and can mask missing salty flavor.

PER SERVING: Calories: 255; Total fat: 9 g; Saturated fat: 1 g; Cholesterol: 55 mg; Sodium: 331 mg; Potassium: 279 mg; Total carbohydrates: 16 g; Fiber: 5 g; Sugars: 6 g; Protein: 26 g

Crispy Walnut Chicken with Steamed Broccoli

This recipe is a healthy version of "shake and bake" chicken, but the high-sodium processed mix is replaced with a mix of ground walnuts and flaxseeds—excellent sources of heart-healthy fats, fiber, vitamins, and minerals. Gluten-free and super fast to prep, the coating ensures the chicken is always moist and juicy. In the last minutes of cooking, simply microwave fiber- and nutrient-rich broccoli for a nutritious low-calorie meal with fewer than ten ingredients.

½ cup chopped walnuts (see Tip)

½ cup flaxseed meal

1 teaspoon sweet paprika

½ teaspoon freshly ground black pepper

⅛ teaspoon salt

4 boneless, skinless chicken breasts (4 ounces each)

4 cups broccoli florets

1 lemon, quartered

1. Preheat the oven to 350°F. Lightly coat a baking dish with cooking spray.

2. In a food processor or blender, process the walnuts into a meal.

3. In a resealable plastic bag, combine the walnut meal, flaxseed meal, paprika, black pepper, and salt. One at a time, place a chicken breast in the bag, seal the bag, and shake until evenly coated. Transfer the coated chicken breast to the prepared baking dish and sprinkle with any remaining walnut/flaxseed meal. (Do not keep the walnut/flaxseed mixture for another purpose as it has touched the raw chicken and you want to avoid cross-contamination.)

4. Transfer the chicken to the oven and bake until no longer pink in the center, the juices run clear, and an instant-read thermometer inserted in the center reads 165°F, 25 to 30 minutes.

5. Meanwhile, about 5 minutes before the chicken is done, place the broccoli in a microwave-safe dish and pour about 4 tablespoons water over the top. Cover with a microwave lid or paper towel and cook on high for 3 minutes. Remove the lid carefully and check to see if the broccoli is tender. If not, microwave in additional 1-minute increments. Carefully remove the broccoli from the microwave and drain.

6. Serve the chicken with the broccoli, with lemon quarters for squeezing. If desired, season the dish with a dash of salt, pepper, and paprika.

TIP: You can use any type of nut in this recipe, as all nuts are very nutritious and rich in essential vitamins, minerals, and fiber. Mixing the nuts with ground flaxseed keeps calories in check while still boosting the nutrient content of the coating. If you already have almond meal/flour on hand for baking, use that for a variation and/or to save prep time.

PER SERVING: Calories: 310; Total fat: 18 g; Saturated fat: 1 g; Cholesterol: 55 mg; Sodium: 308 mg; Potassium: 407 mg; Total carbohydrates: 14 g; Fiber: 8 g; Sugars: 2 g; Protein: 31 g

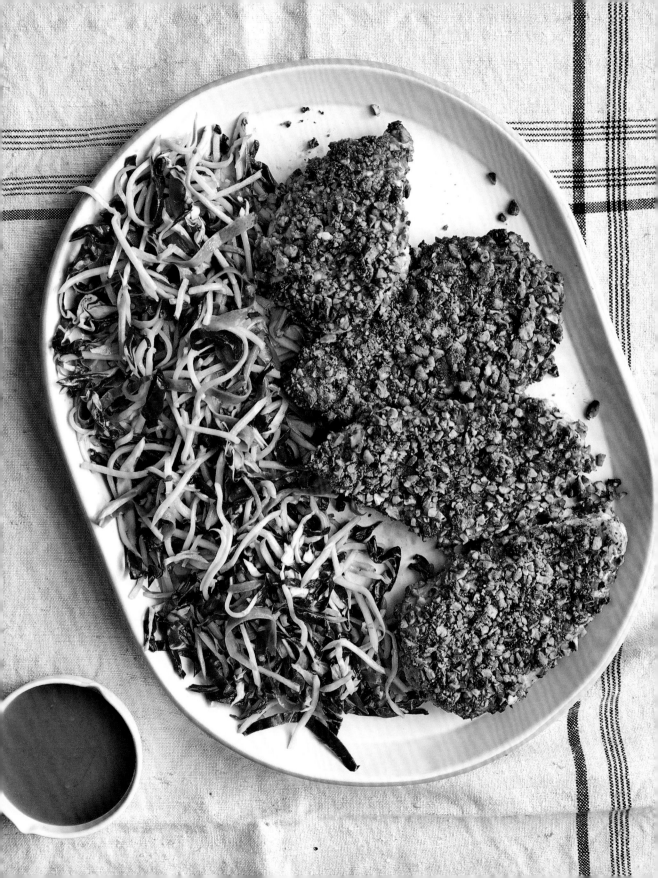

Pistachio-Crusted Honey-Mustard Turkey Cutlets and Radicchio Slaw

Consider keeping a stock of pistachio nuts on hand in your pantry, as you can eat more pistachios per serving than any other kind of nut. A serving of 30 pistachios has just 100 calories and their unique flavor makes them perfect for adding to smoothies, salads, and as a healthy fiber-, vitamin-, and mineral-rich coating in place of bread crumbs in savory recipes. In this quick and easy recipe, pistachios are used as a crust for protein-rich turkey, which is pared with a crunchy radicchio slaw.

1 cup unsalted pistachios

½ teaspoon freshly ground black pepper

⅛ teaspoon salt

½ teaspoon sweet paprika

¼ cup honey

¼ cup Dijon mustard

1 teaspoon fresh lime juice

2 tablespoons extra-virgin olive oil

1 large egg

4 turkey breast cutlets (4 ounces each), such as Honeysuckle White (see Tip, page 158)

1 cup thinly sliced radicchio

1 cup broccoli slaw

2 medium carrots, cut into ribbons with a vegetable peeler

1. Preheat the oven to 400°F. Line a large baking sheet with parchment paper.

2. In a high-powered blender or food processor, combine the pistachios, black pepper, salt, and paprika and pulse a few times until the mixture is crumbly but before it forms a paste, 20 to 30 seconds. Transfer the mixture to a large shallow dish.

3. In a small bowl, combine the honey, mustard, lime juice, and olive oil and whisk to combine. Reserve half of the mixture for dressing the radicchio slaw and pour the remaining half into a separate shallow bowl and whisk in the egg until well combined.

4. Working with one cutlet at a time, coat with a thin layer of the egg/mustard mixture, gently shaking off the excess, then coat on both sides with the pistachio mixture, gently shaking off excess. Place the cutlets on the lined baking sheet.

5. Transfer to the oven and bake for 8 minutes, then carefully flip and continue baking until the cutlets are slightly browned and crispy, for an additional 8 to 10 minutes.

6. Meanwhile, in a medium bowl, combine the radicchio, broccoli slaw, and carrot ribbons. Drizzle the reserved honey-mustard mixture over the slaw and toss to coat.

7. Serve the cutlets with the radicchio slaw.

PER SERVING: Calories: 468; Total fat: 22 g; Saturated fat: 3 g; Cholesterol: 123 mg; Sodium: 534 mg; Potassium: 463 mg; Total carbohydrates: 31 g; Fiber: 5 g; Sugars: 21 g; Protein: 36 g

Lemongrass Coconut Curry Chicken

This flavorful, quick, and easy recipe takes a traditionally high-calorie and high-fat dish and modifies it with a few healthful change-ups so you have another delicious option to choose from on your DASH weight-loss plan. High-fat and high-calorie coconut milk is switched for light, while the oil is reduced and the seasonings are increased. With all of the classic tastes of your favorite coconut curry chicken, this recipe is high in appetite-squashing lean protein, fiber, vitamins, and minerals.

1 cup brown jasmine rice

2 teaspoons extra-virgin olive oil

3 cloves garlic, minced

1 medium red bell pepper, sliced

3 tablespoons minced fresh ginger

1½ tablespoons curry powder

1 stalk lemongrass (see Tip), bottom 6 inches only, outer leaves peeled

1 tablespoon honey

2/3 cup canned "lite" coconut milk

3/4 cup low-sodium chicken broth

1 pound boneless, skinless chicken breasts, cut into bite-size cubes

1/4 cup chopped unsalted cashews

2 tablespoons unsweetened shredded coconut (optional)

2 tablespoons golden raisins

4 tablespoons chopped fresh cilantro leaves

1. In a medium saucepan with a tight-fitting lid, combine the rice and 2 cups water, bring to a boil, stir once, cover, and reduce the heat to low. Simmer until all of the liquid is absorbed, 30 to 35 minutes. Do not lift the lid or stir during cooking.

2. Meanwhile, in a large skillet, heat the olive oil over medium-high heat. Add the garlic and sauté for 1 minute. Add the bell pepper and continue cooking for 2 minutes. Add the ginger and curry powder and mix well, cooking for 1 minute.

3. Mash the lemongrass lightly with a kitchen mallet to release the flavors. Add the lemongrass, honey, coconut milk, and broth to the skillet, reduce the heat to medium, and cook for 3 minutes, until the ingredients are combined and simmering.

4. Add the chicken to the pan, stir all of the ingredients, and cover the pan. Simmer over medium-low heat until the chicken is cooked through, about 25 to 30 minutes.

5. Remove and discard the lemongrass stalk and stir in the cashews, shredded coconut (if using), raisins, and cilantro.

6. Fluff the rice with a fork and portion onto 4 serving plates. Serve the chicken over the rice.

TIP: Lemongrass can be found with the other fresh herbs in the grocery store and adds a really nice touch of citrusy flavor. If you can't find it, substitute the zest from 1 lemon.

PER SERVING: Calories: 426; Total fat: 12 g; Saturated fat: 5 g; Cholesterol: 55 mg; Sodium: 229 mg; Potassium: 153 mg; Total carbohydrates: 52 g; Fiber: 5 g; Sugars: 8 g; Protein: 29 g

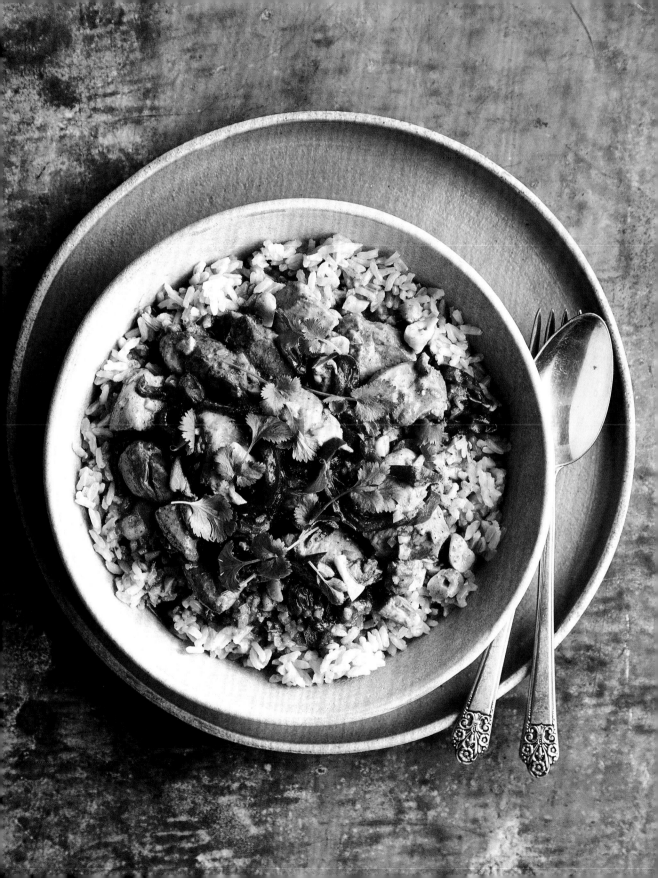

Pan-Seared Turkey Cutlets and Pepper Sauté

Turkey breast is an excellent source of lean, low-calorie protein, and is high in essential B vitamins, potassium, and iron. Boneless, skinless turkey breast cutlets cook up quickly, and since this recipe uses just one pan and a handful of pantry ingredients, you can have a healthy dinner on the table in minutes with minimal cleanup. Slightly crispy on the outside and juicy on the inside, the use of tarragon complements the flavors of this turkey dish nicely.

Salt and freshly ground black pepper

1 pound turkey breast cutlets (see Tip)

2 tablespoons extra-virgin olive oil

2 cloves garlic, minced

1 large yellow bell pepper, cut into strips

1 large red bell pepper, cut into strips

1 cup button mushrooms, sliced

1 tablespoon dried tarragon

1 (14.5-ounce) can no-salt-added diced tomatoes, undrained

TIP: Honeysuckle White is one brand of turkey breast cutlet you can look for. Their turkeys are raised without growth-promoting hormones. The cutlets should be available in most grocery stores in the meat department.

1. Sprinkle a dash of salt and pepper over the turkey cutlets. In a large skillet, heat 1 tablespoon of the olive oil over medium-high heat. Add the turkey cutlets to the skillet and cook until browned on the bottom, 1 to 3 minutes. Flip and continue cooking until cooked all the way through, 1 to 3 minutes more. The outside should be nicely browned and the inside fully cooked and opaque throughout. Remove the turkey to a plate and cover with foil to keep warm.

2. Add the remaining 1 tablespoon olive oil to the skillet, then add the garlic and sauté for 1 minute, until sizzling. Add the bell peppers and mushrooms and continue cooking until starting to soften, 5 to 7 minutes.

3. Add the tarragon and tomatoes and their juices, cover, and bring to a simmer, stirring often, 3 to 5 minutes, until slightly reduced.

4. Return the turkey cutlets to the skillet and bring to a simmer. Reduce the heat to medium-low and cook for 2 to 3 minutes to warm the turkey through.

PER SERVING: Calories: 225; Total fat: 8 g; Saturated fat: 1 g; Cholesterol: 70 mg; Sodium: 67 mg; Potassium: 180 mg; Total carbohydrates: 10 g; Fiber: 2 g; Sugars: 3 g; Protein: 30 g

PREP TIME: 10 MINUTES · COOK TIME: 15 MINUTES · SERVES 4

Oatmeal-Crusted Chicken Tenders

These healthy oatmeal-crusted chicken tenders are kid-approved, easy to make, deliciously crispy on the outside, and juicy on the inside. Coating the tenders in oatmeal instead of bread crumbs adds valuable heart-healthy fiber and B vitamins while baking reduces the need for added fats. High in satiating protein with added calcium from the cheese, these homemade chicken tenders make a great snack, appetizer, and healthy dinner. Serve with a side of green vegetables and maybe a dipping sauce (see Tips).

1 cup rolled oats (see Tips)

½ cup freshly grated Parmesan cheese

2 teaspoons chopped fresh rosemary

⅛ teaspoon sweet paprika

⅛ teaspoon salt

¼ teaspoon freshly ground black pepper

1 pound boneless, skinless chicken tenders

TIPS: For a variation, try a different type of flaked grain such as barley flakes or quinoa flakes.

The tenders freeze well, so consider baking a double batch so you have something healthy on hand on days when you just have too much to do.

For a healthy dip, try serving these with Herbed Greek Yogurt Dressing (page 201), Black Bean Mango Salsa (page 196), your favorite mustard, or ketchup.

1. Preheat the oven to 450°F. Lightly coat a large baking sheet with cooking spray.

2. Place the oats in a food processor or blender and pulse for 30 seconds until coarsely ground. You do not need the oatmeal to be powdered, just a few pulses to break it down. Add the Parmesan, rosemary, paprika, salt, and pepper and pulse to combine. Pour into a shallow bowl.

3. Place each chicken tender between two sheets of plastic wrap and use a meat mallet or small heavy skillet to pound to a ¼-inch thickness. Coat both sides of the tenders with cooking spray, then dredge the tenders in the oat mixture.

4. Place the tenders on the prepared baking sheet and bake until browned and crispy, turning at the halfway point, about 15 minutes.

PER SERVING: Calories: 225; Total fat: 6 g; Saturated fat: 2 g; Cholesterol: 70 mg; Sodium: 493 mg; Potassium: 2 mg; Total carbohydrates: 14 g; Fiber: 2 g; Sugars: <1 g; Protein: 30 g

Fresh Rosemary Balsamic Chicken and Brussels Sprouts with Toasted Almonds

This healthy, light, and flavorful recipe uses balsamic vinegar to make a low-sodium reduction sauce with garlic and fresh rosemary to give the chicken a wonderful taste. Rich in health-promoting polyphenols and antioxidants, balsamic vinegar promotes healthy cholesterol levels and may be beneficial for blood pressure. Dark in color with a sweet, pungent taste, balsamic is also used to bring out the sweetness in the Brussels sprouts, which are roasted and topped with toasted almonds.

CHICKEN

½ cup + 2 tablespoons balsamic vinegar

1 teaspoon extra-virgin olive oil

1 tablespoon chopped fresh rosemary

1 clove garlic, minced

⅛ teaspoon salt

Freshly ground black pepper

2 boneless, skinless chicken breasts (4 ounces each)

BRUSSELS SPROUTS

½ pound Brussels sprouts, trimmed of outer leaves and halved lengthwise

2 teaspoons extra-virgin olive oil

2 teaspoons balsamic vinegar

⅛ teaspoon salt

⅛ teaspoon freshly ground black pepper

2 tablespoons sliced almonds

Sprigs fresh rosemary

1. Marinate the chicken: In a small saucepan, combine the balsamic vinegar, olive oil, rosemary, garlic, salt, and pepper. Bring to a boil, reduce the heat to medium, and simmer until reduced by half, about 3 minutes. Place in the refrigerator to cool for 15 minutes or for a quicker chill, place in the freezer for 5 minutes.

2. Coat a 9 × 9-inch baking dish with cooking spray. Place the chicken in the baking dish and pour the cooled marinade over it. Marinate in the refrigerator for 30 minutes.

3. Preheat the oven to 375°F.

4. When the chicken is done marinating, remove from the refrigerator and cover the baking dish with foil.

5. Prepare the Brussels sprouts: In a medium bowl, toss the Brussels sprouts with the olive oil, balsamic vinegar, salt, and pepper. Spread on a nonstick baking sheet.

6. Transfer the chicken and Brussels sprouts to the oven and roast until an instant-read thermometer inserted in a chicken breast reads 165°F and the Brussels sprouts are browned and tender, 30 to 35 minutes. Turn the Brussels sprouts once about halfway through cooking.

7. While the chicken and Brussels sprouts cook, in a small dry skillet, toast the almonds over medium heat, stirring constantly, until golden and fragrant, 3 to 4 minutes.

8. Remove the Brussels and chicken from the oven, mix the almonds with the sprouts, and garnish with rosemary sprigs to serve.

PER SERVING: Calories: 304; Total fat: 12 g; Saturated fat: 1 g; Cholesterol: 55 mg; Sodium: 556 mg; Potassium: 449 mg; Total carbohydrates: 23 g; Fiber: 5 g; Sugars: 3 g; Protein: 28 g

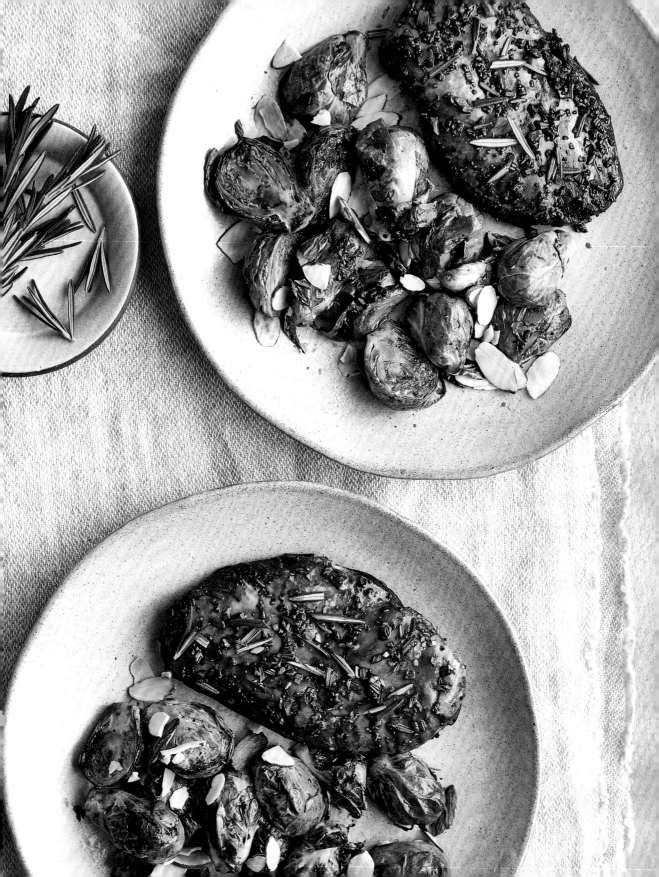

Slow Cooker Pineapple Chicken

A slow cooker is a wonderful appliance for busy folks wishing to eat healthy. Just prep on a busy weekend morning and have a nutritious, satisfying dinner. This refreshing and tropical pineapple chicken recipe is full of vitamin C from the pineapple and peppers with ample amounts of lean, high-quality protein to keep you feeling full. Low in sodium, and calories with minimal fats, this is a nourishing nutrient-rich dinner the whole family will enjoy. Serve in lettuce leaves or over brown rice or another whole grain or riced cauliflower.

1 pound frozen boneless, skinless chicken breasts

2 medium carrots, sliced

1 medium red bell pepper, cut into 1-inch chunks

1 (20-ounce) can water- or juice-packed crushed or chopped pineapple, undrained

¼ cup balsamic vinegar

1 tablespoon reduced-sodium soy sauce (see Tip)

2 tablespoons pure maple syrup

1 teaspoon red pepper flakes

TIP: Coconut aminos is a gluten-free lower-sodium soy sauce alternative that would work great in this recipe and be a healthy addition to your pantry staples. Coconut aminos are made from coconut sap with a rich, dark, salty, and slightly sweet flavor.

1. Coat the inside of the slow cooker with cooking spray. Add the chicken, carrots, and bell pepper.

2. Drain the pineapple juice from the can into a small bowl. Add the balsamic vinegar, soy sauce, maple syrup, and pepper flakes and whisk to combine. Pour over the chicken and add the crushed or chopped pineapple.

3. Cover the slow cooker and cook on LOW for 4 to 5 hours or on HIGH for 1½ to 2 hours, until cooked through. The vegetables should be fork-tender and the chicken should register 165°F on an instant-read thermometer and be tender enough to easily tear apart with a fork. Remove the chicken from the slow cooker and shred with two forks. Return the chicken to the slow cooker, stir to mix the ingredients, and set the temperature to warm until ready to serve.

PER SERVING: Calories: 242; Total fat: 2 g; Saturated fat: 0 g; Cholesterol: 55 mg; Sodium: 376 mg; Potassium: 307 mg; Total carbohydrates: 34 g; Fiber: 2 g; Sugars: 27 g; Protein: 24 g

Roasted Cajun Blackened Salmon with Asparagus

Many people are tentative about cooking salmon at home, but it's really easy to do with this quick and simple recipe. A blend of savory, spicy, and sweet, Cajun seasonings are used as a coating for the fish, which is baked up to crispy blackened perfection in just minutes. While the salmon bakes, fiber- and nutrient-rich asparagus is roasted and used as a side with amazing taste to make a complete meal—perfect for any night of the week.

2 teaspoons dried parsley

1 teaspoon ground cumin

1 teaspoon garlic powder

1 teaspoon onion powder

1 teaspoon sweet paprika

1 teaspoon dark brown sugar

¼ teaspoon chili powder

¼ teaspoon salt, plus more to taste

¼ teaspoon freshly ground black pepper, plus more to taste

4 skinless salmon fillets (6 ounces each); see Tip

1 pound asparagus, tough ends trimmed

1 tablespoon extra-virgin olive oil

1 lemon, quartered

1. Preheat the oven to 425°F. Line two large baking sheets with foil and lightly coat with cooking spray.

2. In a shallow bowl, combine the parsley, cumin, garlic powder, onion powder, paprika, brown sugar, chili powder, and ¼ teaspoon each salt and black pepper and mix the blackened seasoning thoroughly.

3. Place the salmon on a plate and coat with cooking spray. Season with 1 teaspoon of the blackened seasoning, flip, coat with more cooking spray and season with another 1 teaspoon of the seasoning. Place on one of the prepared baking sheets.

4. Place the asparagus in a small bowl and drizzle with the olive oil and sprinkle with salt and pepper, if desired. Place on the second prepared baking sheet.

5. Transfer the salmon and asparagus to the oven and roast until the asparagus is tender and slightly browned and the salmon flakes easily with a fork, is blackened and crispy on the outside, and an instant-read thermometer reads 145°F, 12 to 15 minutes, depending on the thickness of the salmon and the asparagus.

6. Portion onto 4 plates and squeeze fresh lemon juice over each.

TIP: Salmon is an excellent source of heart-healthy omega-3 fatty acids and the American Heart Association recommends aiming to include at least two servings per week for heart health. There is a very big price range among the various types of salmon fillets, but they are all healthy, so choose the salmon you can afford. Pink and chum are smaller fish, but are very budget friendly.

PER SERVING: Calories: 280; Total fat: 11 g; Saturated fat: 2 g; Cholesterol: 75 mg; Sodium: 227 mg; Potassium: 369 mg; Total carbohydrates: 10 g; Fiber: 4 g; Sugars: 3 g; Protein: 38 g

Orange-Thyme Salmon and Summer Squash in a Packet

This delicious main dish can be prepped and refrigerated ahead of cooking and then placed in the oven when you are ready. All of the ingredients go into the packet (see Tip), which allows the fish and vegetables to steam in their own juices, locking in aroma and flavor. With no dishes to clean, and individually portioned, this recipe makes it super simple to have a heart-healthy, low-calorie meal on the table within minutes.

Juice of 1 lemon

1 tablespoon extra-virgin olive oil

2 teaspoons dried thyme

¼ teaspoon salt

¼ teaspoon freshly ground black pepper

2 cups sliced yellow summer squash (about 2 medium)

2 cups sliced zucchini (about 2 medium)

1 small red onion, thinly sliced

2 blood oranges, peeled and thinly sliced

4 skinless salmon fillets (6 ounces each)

4 sprigs fresh thyme

1. Preheat the oven to 400°F. Tear off 4 pieces of foil or parchment that are 2 inches longer than the salmon fillets.

2. In a medium bowl, combine the lemon juice, olive oil, dried thyme, salt, and pepper.

3. Place the foil/parchment pieces on your work surface and on one side of each piece of foil/parchment, layer one-quarter of the yellow squash, zucchini, red onion, and blood orange. Top each stack of vegetables with a salmon fillet and drizzle each stack with the lemon juice mixture. Place a thyme sprig on top of each piece of fish.

4. Fold the other half of the foil/parchment over the ingredients. To seal the packets, begin at one corner and tightly fold the edges over about ½ inch all around, overlapping the folds. The foil/parchment should not come undone.

5. Place the packets on a baking sheet. Transfer to the oven and bake until the salmon turns opaque throughout, about 20 minutes.

6. Serve the pouches on a plate or remove the contents to a plate, being very careful of the escaping steam when opening as it will be very hot. Spoon any liquid remaining in the foil/parchment over the salmon and vegetables.

TIP: Packet cooking is a great technique for the novice and seasoned fish cook alike. A fuss-free, foolproof method, cooking in a packet keeps your fish juicy and the house from smelling like fish. You can use parchment or foil and bake the packets in the oven or on the grill. Packet cooking also works well with chicken, turkey, tofu, and vegetables.

PER SERVING: Calories: 309; Total fat: 11 g; Saturated fat: 2 g; Cholesterol: 75 mg; Sodium: 279 mg; Potassium: 615 mg; Total carbohydrates: 18 g; Fiber: 6 g; Sugars: 10 g; Protein: 37 g

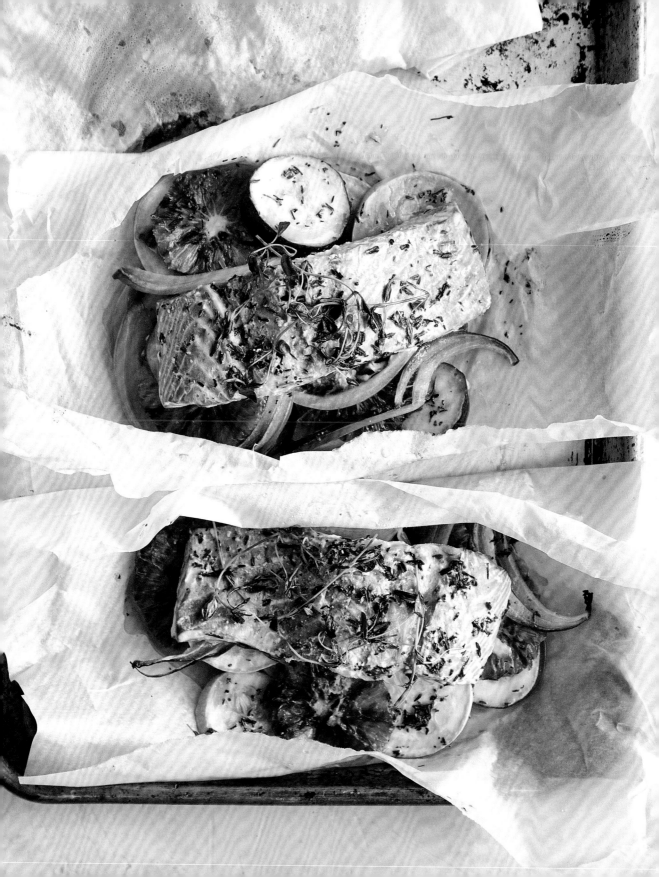

One-Pot Shrimp Pasta Primavera

Low in calories yet full of flavor and loaded with lean protein and ample amounts of fiber-rich vegetables and a serving of whole grains, this dish comes together in just minutes with a handful of ingredients. "Primavera" in a recipe title indicates a mixture of fresh vegetables, so feel free to use your favorites or what is available and in season in this recipe.

8 ounces whole-grain angel hair pasta (see Tip)

2 tablespoons extra-virgin olive oil

2 tablespoons minced garlic

1 cup broccoli florets

1 large red bell pepper, chopped

1 cup sliced yellow squash (about 1 medium)

1 cup green peas (if frozen, slightly thawed)

8 ounces frozen peeled and deveined cooked shrimp

2 teaspoons dried basil

2 teaspoons dried oregano

¼ teaspoon red pepper flakes

Salt and freshly ground black pepper (optional)

1 lemon, halved

4 tablespoons grated Parmesan cheese

1. Cook the pasta according to the package directions. Drain and cover to keep warm.

2. In a large nonstick skillet, heat the olive oil over medium heat. Add the garlic and sauté for 1 minute. Add the broccoli, bell pepper, and squash and sauté until crisp-tender, 3 to 4 minutes.

3. Add the peas and shrimp and sauté until just heated through. Season with the basil, oregano, pepper flakes, and salt and black pepper, if desired. Squeeze the lemon over the shrimp and vegetables. Continue to cook for 2 to 3 minutes, until the liquid has been reduced by half. Remove from the heat.

4. Toss the shrimp and vegetables with the pasta. Portion onto 4 plates and top each serving with 1 tablespoon Parmesan.

TIP: There is a dizzying array of pastas to choose from these days, but you want one made with whole grains, as whole grains are high in fiber, which contributes to satiety, or that feeling of fullness. Bean pastas make an outstanding choice with varieties made from lentils, black beans, chickpeas, and even adzuki beans. Gluten-free pastas tend to be very low in fiber and nutrients in general, so only choose gluten-free if you have celiac or a gluten sensitivity.

PER SERVING: Calories: 405; Total fat: 11 g; Saturated fat: 2 g; Cholesterol: 115 mg; Sodium: 243 mg; Potassium: 388 mg; Total carbohydrates: 54 g; Fiber: 10 g; Sugars: 5 g; Protein: 24 g

Haddock Tacos with Cabbage Slaw

This simple and quick fish taco recipe features the saltwater fish haddock, a popular fish low in calories and high in protein, B vitamins, and the minerals magnesium and selenium. With a firm, white flesh and a mild flavor, this is a perfect choice for those who find the taste of salmon too strong. Cooked quickly on the stovetop with Mexican spices, this meal provides you with lean protein, healthy fats from avocado, fruits, vegetables, and whole grains.

1 teaspoon ground cumin

½ teaspoon chili powder

⅛ teaspoon salt

⅛ teaspoon freshly ground black pepper

8 ounces skinless haddock fillets, cut into 1-inch chunks (see Tip)

2 cups angel hair cabbage

½ avocado, chopped

2 tablespoons fresh lime juice

3 teaspoons extra-virgin olive oil

2 (6-inch) whole-wheat tortillas, warmed

Fresh cilantro

1. In a small bowl, combine the cumin, chili powder, salt, and pepper. Add the haddock and toss to coat.

2. In a separate small bowl, mix together the cabbage, avocado, lime juice, and 1 teaspoon of the olive oil.

3. In a medium skillet, heat the remaining 2 teaspoons olive oil over medium-high heat. Add the haddock and cook, turning, until the fish is just opaque and flakes easily with a fork, 4 to 5 minutes.

4. Divide the fish between the warmed tortillas and top with the cabbage avocado mixture. Serve garnished with fresh cilantro.

TIP: You can use any type of whitefish in this recipe, such as flounder, which is another mild, whitefish and a heart-healthy choice.

PER SERVING: Calories: 368; Total fat: 16 g; Saturated fat: 2 g; Cholesterol: 84 mg; Sodium: 408 mg; Potassium: 261 mg; Total carbohydrates: 22 g; Fiber: 7 g; Sugars: 2 g; Protein: 32 g

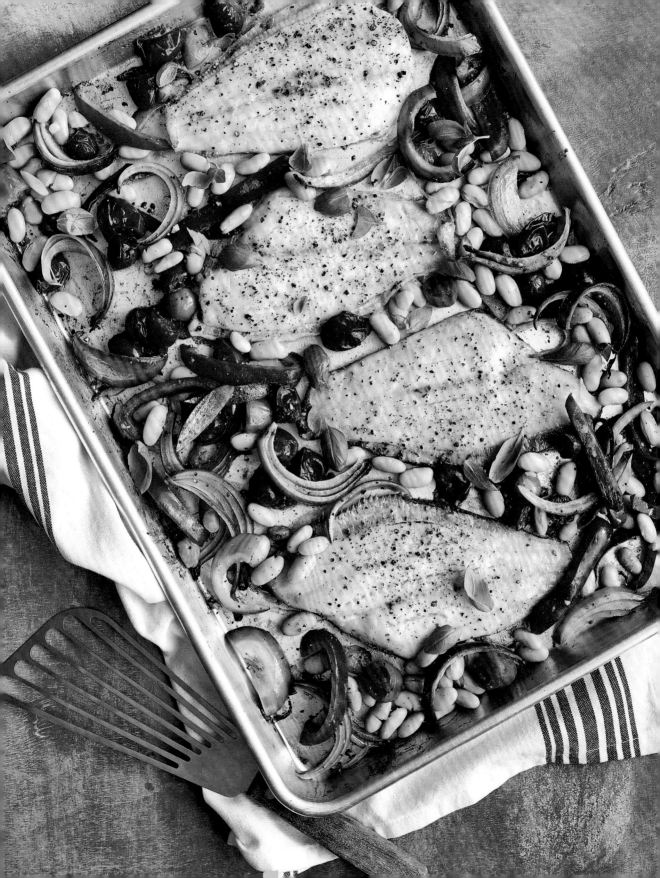

Sheet Pan Flounder with White Beans, Tomatoes, and Basil

Sheet pan dinners are perfect for the busy cook, and this recipe includes all of the essential elements of a DASH weight-loss recipe: Lean whitefish provides low-calorie, high-quality protein; white beans provide fiber, plant protein, and B vitamins; tomatoes add blood-pressure-lowering potassium and antioxidants; and basil provides disease-protective plant chemicals and reduces the need for added salt. Quick, easy, healthy, requires minimal fuss, and delicious—everything you want in a recipe!

2 (15-ounce) cans cannellini beans or other white bean, rinsed and drained

1 medium red onion, sliced

1 large red bell pepper, sliced

1 pint cherry tomatoes, halved (a pint of mixed colors provides a striking dish)

4 cloves garlic, minced

2 teaspoons dried marjoram

2 tablespoons extra-virgin olive oil

Salt and freshly ground black pepper

¼ cup white wine

4 flounder fillets (4 ounces each)

1 lemon, halved

4 tablespoons coarsely chopped fresh basil

TIP: You can vary the recipe by swapping out the white beans for chickpeas or black beans and replacing the seasonings with paprika, cumin, and cilantro for garnish. You could also swap out the red bell pepper for jarred roasted red pepper.

1. Preheat the oven to 400°F. Line a rimmed baking sheet with foil.

2. Spread the beans, onion, and bell pepper over the baking sheet and nestle the cherry tomatoes cut side up among them. Sprinkle with half of the minced garlic and all the marjoram. Drizzle with 1 tablespoon of the olive oil and season with a dash each of salt and black pepper. Transfer to the oven and roast for 10 minutes.

3. Remove the baking sheet from the oven and drizzle with the white wine. Move the vegetables to the sides and place the flounder on the baking sheet. Sprinkle with the remaining garlic and 1 tablespoon olive oil. Season lightly with salt and pepper, if desired, and squeeze the lemon over the top. Roast until the fish is cooked through, opaque, and flakes easily with a fork, about 15 minutes.

4. Place a fillet on each of 4 serving plates. Portion the vegetables onto the plates and sprinkle each serving with 1 tablespoon fresh basil.

PER SERVING: Calories: 368; Total fat: 8 g; Saturated fat: 1 g; Cholesterol: 65 mg; Sodium: 89 mg; Potassium: 316 mg; Total carbohydrates: 40 g; Fiber: 10 g; Sugars: 3 g; Protein: 32 g

Lemon-Ginger Cod with Roasted Cauliflower and Carrots

Cod is another great protein pick with its low calorie count and mild taste. A good source of protein, phosphorus, healthy B vitamins, and omega-3 fats, cod is paired in this recipe with whole-grain brown rice and perfectly seasoned roasted vegetables for a gourmet-tasting meal that takes minimal time to prepare.

6 medium carrots, sliced

3 cups or about 1 medium head cauliflower, trimmed into small florets

3 tablespoons extra-virgin olive oil

Salt and freshly ground pepper

2 cups instant brown rice (see Tip)

1 tablespoon grated fresh ginger

2 cloves garlic, grated

2 lemons, sliced

4 cod fillets (4 ounces each)

½ cup dry white wine

¼ cup chopped fresh chives, plus more for garnish

1. Preheat the oven to 400°F. Coat a rimmed baking sheet with cooking spray.

2. Arrange the vegetables on the baking sheet and drizzle with 1 tablespoon of the olive oil and, if desired, lightly season with salt and pepper. Bake until tender and golden brown, about 25 minutes.

3. Meanwhile cook the rice according to the package directions.

4. In a small bowl, combine 1 tablespoon of the olive oil, the ginger, garlic, lemon slices, and salt and pepper, if desired. Set aside.

5. In a large skillet, heat the remaining 1 tablespoon olive oil over medium-high heat. When the oil is shimmering, add the fish and sear for 5 minutes, then move to the side leaving extra room in the pan. Add the ginger/garlic/lemon slice mixture to the pan and sauté until the lemon slices have turned golden brown, 3 to 4 minutes.

6. Add the white wine and chives and cook until a sauce begins to form, about 3 minutes. Scoop some of the sauce over the fish.

7. Add the cooked rice to the pan and simmer until the sauce is fully absorbed, 3 to 5 minutes.

8. Place a cod fillet on each of 4 serving plates. Portion the rice and sauce mixture next to the fish. Remove the vegetables from the oven and portion onto each plate. Garnish with additional chives, if desired.

TIP: You may be surprised to learn that instant brown rice is a healthy choice. The nutritional differences between a serving of long-grain brown, which requires 35 to 45 minutes to cook, and instant brown rice, which cooks in 5 minutes, are insignificant. Instant rice has simply been cooked and dehydrated so that it cooks more quickly than regular brown rice.

PER SERVING: Calories: 450; Total fat: 13 g; Saturated fat: 2 g; Cholesterol: 62 mg; Sodium: 187 mg; Potassium: 959 mg; Total carbohydrates: 53 g; Fiber: 9 g; Sugars: 6 g; Protein: 32 g

Lemon-Garlic Tilapia with Roasted Vegetables and Arugula

Tilapia is a budget-friendly fish that is an excellent source of lean, high-quality protein. A mild, lean white fish, tilapia boasts healthful omega-3 fatty acids, B vitamins, iron, vitamin D, and selenium. For this quick and easy one-pan dish, tilapia is roasted with fiber- and nutrient-rich broccoli and summer squash and paired with a peppery arugula salad.

3 cups broccoli florets

1 cup sliced yellow squash (about 1 medium)

2 tablespoons + 2 teaspoons extra-virgin olive oil

Salt and freshly ground black pepper

2 tablespoons fresh lemon juice

2 tablespoons minced shallot

2 tablespoons chopped fresh parsley

1 tablespoon minced garlic

4 tilapia fillets (4 ounces each)

5 ounces baby arugula

2 tablespoons grated Parmesan cheese

TIP: You can enjoy this dish on its own, or for a speedy supper, serve with instant brown rice, quinoa, whole-wheat couscous, or crusty whole-grain bread.

1. Preheat the oven to 400°F. Coat a rimmed baking sheet with cooking spray.

2. Place the broccoli and squash on the baking sheet, drizzle with 1 tablespoon of the olive oil and season with salt and pepper, if desired. Push the vegetables to the sides of the pan.

3. In a small bowl, mix together 1 tablespoon of the olive oil, the lemon juice, shallot, parsley, garlic, ¼ teaspoon pepper, and ⅛ teaspoon salt. Place the tilapia fillets on the baking sheet in between the vegetables and season with the lemon/shallot/parsley mixture, gently pressing into the fish, turning, and seasoning the other side.

4. Transfer the baking sheet to the oven and bake until the fish flakes easily with a fork, 12 to 15 minutes.

5. Meanwhile, in a medium bowl, toss together the arugula, remaining 2 teaspoons olive oil, the Parmesan, and salt and pepper, if desired. Toss to combine.

6. Place a tilapia fillet on each of 4 plates. Portion the roasted vegetables and the arugula salad onto the plates.

PER SERVING: Calories: 244; Total fat: 13 g; Saturated fat: 2 g; Cholesterol: 57 mg; Sodium: 208 mg; Potassium: 828 mg; Total carbohydrates: 9 g; Fiber: 3 g; Sugars: 3 g; Protein: 29 g

Easy Scallop Quinoa Paella

Paella is a traditional Spanish dish in which rice—a type similar to that used for risotto—is combined with seafood and/or chicken and seasoned with saffron and other spices. I created this version using one of my favorite grains, quinoa, along with traditional paella ingredients (including fiber-rich green peas and low-calorie and protein-rich scallops), and I substituted turmeric for the more expensive saffron. One of my dad's favorites, this filling dish is made in one pan, is ready in less than 40 minutes, and is full of paella flavor.

1 tablespoon extra-virgin olive oil

1 cup chopped onion

3 cloves garlic, minced

1 medium red bell pepper, chopped

1 cup chopped baby bella mushrooms (5 to 6 mushrooms)

1 (14.5-ounce) can no-salt-added diced tomatoes, undrained

1 (14.5-ounce) can water-packed artichoke hearts, drained and rinsed

1 cup quinoa, rinsed

1 teaspoon smoked paprika

1 teaspoon ground turmeric (see Tip)

Salt and freshly ground black pepper (optional)

2 cups low-sodium vegetable broth

1 cup frozen green peas, thawed

1 pound scallops

1 lemon, halved

Fresh parsley

1. In a large skillet, heat the olive oil over medium heat. Add the onions and garlic and cook until translucent, 3 to 4 minutes. Add the bell pepper and mushrooms and sauté until they start to soften and the mushrooms begin to brown, an additional 3 to 4 minutes.

2. Add the tomatoes and their juices, the artichoke hearts, quinoa, smoked paprika, turmeric, and salt and black pepper, if desired, mixing well to combine. Add the broth and stir again to incorporate. Bring the mixture to a boil, then cover, reduce the heat, and simmer until most of the liquid has been absorbed, about 15 minutes.

3. Add the peas and scallops, cover, and continue cooking until the scallops are cooked through, about 5 minutes.

4. Remove the lid and squeeze the lemon over the top. Serve garnished with fresh parsley.

PER SERVING: Calories: 431; Total fat: 8 g; Saturated fat: <1 g; Cholesterol: 37 mg; Sodium: 339 mg; Potassium: 913 mg; Total carbohydrates: 62 g; Fiber: 15 g; Sugars: 10 g; Protein: 31 g

TIP: If you can find saffron, use that in place of the turmeric for a traditional Spanish flavor. Be sure to rub the threads to release the flavor. Saffron is expensive, so only choose this if your budget allows.

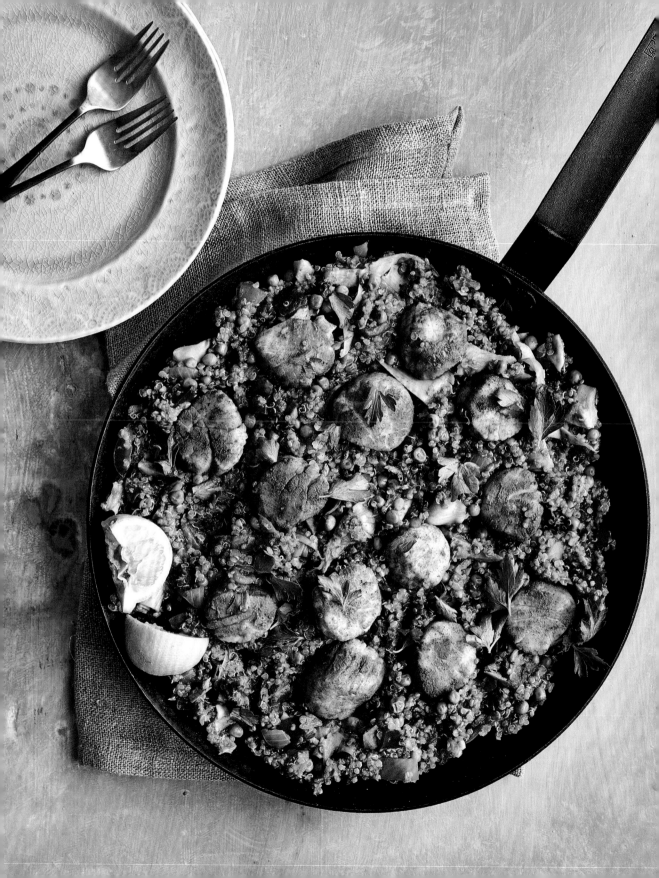

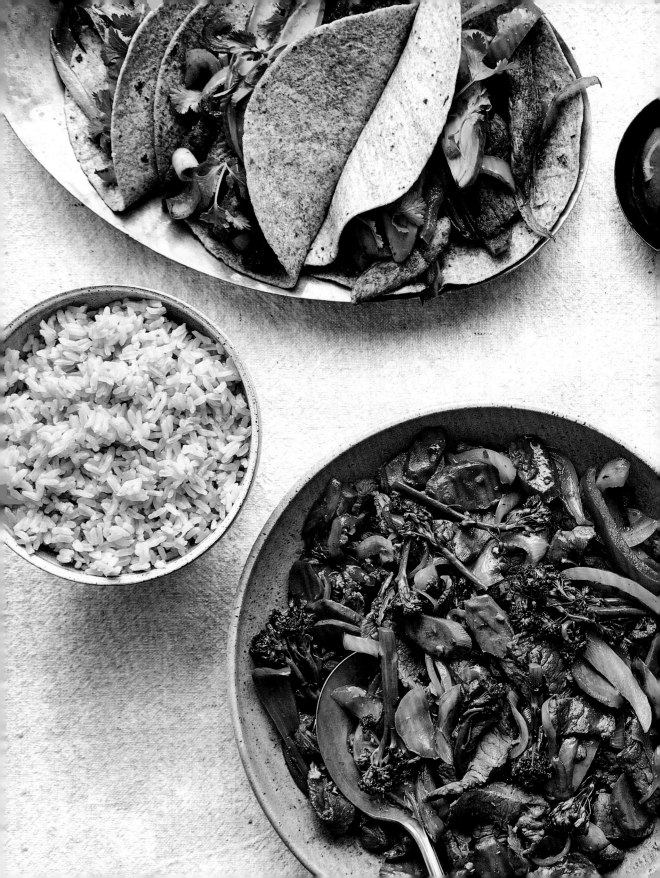

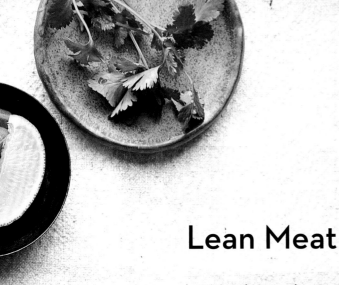

Lean Meat

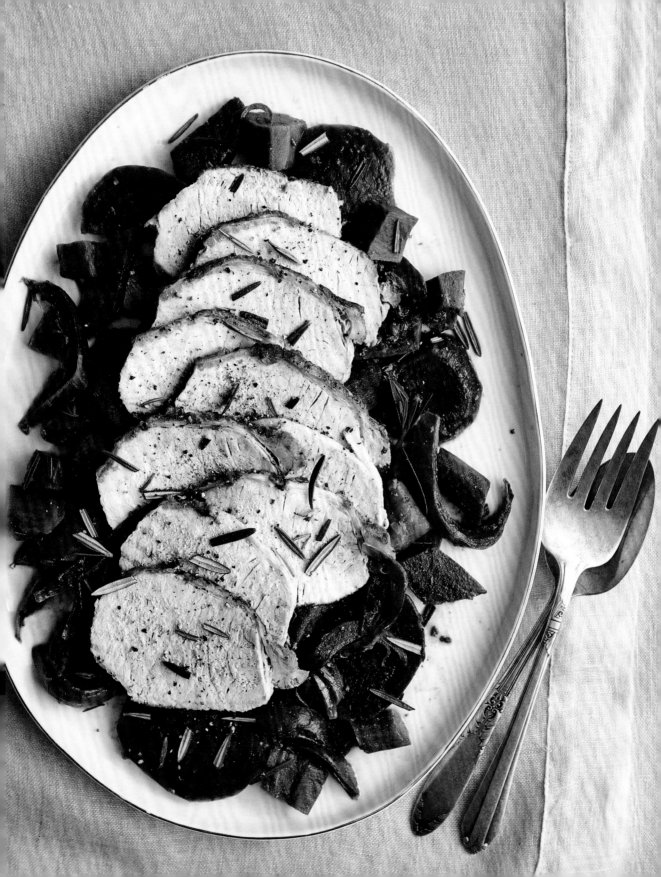

Slow Cooker Rosemary Pork and Root Vegetables

This easy-to-prep pork loin recipe combines the sweet taste of slow-cooked root vegetables with savory pork. Slow-cooking the beets, sweet potatoes, carrots, and parsnips with fragrant rosemary makes them melt-in-the-mouth tender, enhances their natural sweetness, and creates a meal that is simply delicious. Just prep the ingredients the night before, turn on your slow cooker when you leave for errands on the weekend, come home to a nutritious and wholesome meal the whole family will love.

2 large beets (about 1 pound), peeled and sliced

2 cups cubed peeled sweet potato

4 large carrots, cut into 1-inch pieces

1 cup sliced parsnips

1 large Vidalia onion, sliced

1 (4-pound) boneless pork loin roast

8 sprigs fresh rosemary

1 cup low-sodium beef broth

TIP: The National Pork Board recommends cooking pork chops, roasts, and tenderloins to an internal temperature between 145°F (medium-rare) and 160°F (medium) followed by a 3-minute rest.

1. Coat the inside of a 6-quart slow cooker with cooking spray or insert a slow cooker liner.

2. Line the bottom of the slow cooker with half of the beets, sweet potato, carrots, parsnips, and onion. Place the pork on top of the vegetables. Lay the rosemary on top of the pork and cover with the remaining beets, sweet potato, carrots, parsnips, and onion. Pour the broth over the pork and vegetables.

3. Cover and cook on LOW for 7 to 8 hours, or until the pork reaches an internal temperature of 160°F (see Tip).

4. Remove the pork from the slow cooker and allow to rest for 3 minutes. Slice and serve with the root vegetables.

PER SERVING: Calories: 393; Total fat: 9 g; Saturated fat: 2 g; Cholesterol: 141 mg; Sodium: 194 mg; Potassium: 1,308 mg; Total carbohydrates: 22 g; Fiber: 5 g; Sugars: 9 g; Protein: 53 g

Cuban-Style Pork and Black Beans

This Cuban-spiced pork tenderloin and black bean recipe is quick to prepare and will give your taste buds an escape to the tropics and fill your kitchen with wonderful aromas. Full of lean, filling protein, fiber, and nutrient-rich beans and vegetables, this recipe makes it delicious and easy to meet your weight-management goals.

PORK

Grated zest and 2 tablespoons of juice of 1 lime

¼ cup orange juice

1 tablespoon + 1 teaspoon extra-virgin olive oil

1 teaspoon ground cumin

1 teaspoon dried oregano

1 teaspoon red pepper flakes

¼ teaspoon salt

1 pound pork tenderloin

BEANS

1 tablespoon extra-virgin olive oil

1 small onion, chopped

1 medium red bell pepper, chopped

2 large Roma (plum) tomatoes, seeded and chopped

1 tablespoon ground cumin

2 teaspoons dried oregano

1 (15-ounce) can black beans, rinsed and drained

½ cup low-sodium chicken broth or water

¼ cup chopped fresh cilantro (optional)

TIP: This dish is hearty and filling enough to serve as is, but you can also serve it over brown rice or another whole grain.

1. Marinate the pork: In a large plastic bag, combine the lime zest, lime juice, orange juice, 1 teaspoon of the olive oil, the cumin, oregano, pepper flakes, and salt. Add the pork and massage to thoroughly coat. Seal and refrigerate for at least 1 hour and up to 24 hours.

2. Reserving the marinade, remove the pork and cut crosswise into 8 slices. In a large skillet, heat the remaining 1 tablespoon olive oil over medium-high heat. Pan-fry the pork slices until browned on one side, 5 to 6 minutes. Flip, pour the reserved marinade over the pork, and continue cooking until no longer pink in the center, 5 to 7 additional minutes. Reduce the heat to low and cover to keep warm while you make the beans.

3. Prepare the beans: In a second skillet, heat the olive oil over medium-high heat, until shimmering. Add the onion and cook until softened, 3 to 4 minutes. Add the bell pepper, tomatoes, cumin, and oregano and continue cooking until the peppers soften, 3 to 4 minutes.

4. Add the beans and broth, bring to a boil, cover, and simmer until most of the liquid is absorbed, an additional 3 to 4 minutes.

5. Serve the beans with the pork and garnish with fresh cilantro, if desired.

PER SERVING: Calories: 310; Total fat: 11 g; Saturated fat: 2 g; Cholesterol: 45 mg; Sodium: 228 mg; Potassium: 214 mg; Total carbohydrates: 25 g; Fiber: 6 g; Sugars: 3 g; Protein: 31 g

Sweet and Savory Apple-Cinnamon Baked Pork Chops

Many cuts of pork are as lean or leaner than chicken, and any cut from the loin, including pork chops, is a lean choice that you can include with confidence in your DASH weight-loss plan. This quick and easy one-dish meal pairs satiating protein and vitamin- and mineral-rich pork chops with sweet apples, a fruit high in cholesterol-lowering fiber. Enjoy this budget-friendly, quick-to-fix, and delicious sweet and savory dish with a side of steamed green vegetables and a baked sweet potato.

2 apples, peeled and sliced

1 teaspoon ground cinnamon

4 boneless pork chops (½ inch thick)

1 medium red onion, halved and thinly sliced

⅛ teaspoon salt

Freshly ground black pepper (optional)

3 tablespoons dark brown sugar

1 tablespoon extra-virgin olive oil

TIP: For a slightly different variation, substitute 100% apple juice or apple cider for the water. Note that doing so will increase the calorie count of the recipe.

1. Preheat the oven to 375° F.

2. Layer the apples in the bottom of a casserole dish. Sprinkle with ½ teaspoon of the cinnamon.

3. Trim the fat from the pork chops. Lay them on top of the apple slices. Layer the pork chops with the onion slices. Sprinkle with the salt and black pepper, if desired.

4. In a small bowl, combine ¾ cup water (see Tip), the brown sugar, and the remaining ½ teaspoon cinnamon. Pour the mixture over the chops. Drizzle with the olive oil.

5. Transfer to the oven and bake, uncovered, until an instant-read thermometer reads 145°F, 30 to 45 minutes. Allow to rest for 3 minutes before serving.

PER SERVING: Calories: 325; Total fat: 16 g; Saturated fat: 5 g; Cholesterol: 66 mg; Sodium: 126 mg; Potassium: 614 mg; Total carbohydrates: 24 g; Fiber: 3 g; Sugars: 17 g; Protein: 24 g

Parmesan Pork Tenderloin

While there are many ways to cook pork tenderloin, this recipe coats lean, low-fat, potassium-rich pork with calcium-rich Parmesan seasoned with rosemary, then bakes the pork to perfection with minimal fuss. For a lovely, light meal, serve the pork with your favorite vegetable sides and a whole grain.

1 small onion, halved and thinly sliced

¼ cup whole-wheat panko bread crumbs (see Tip)

¼ cup grated Parmesan cheese

2 small cloves garlic, minced

1 teaspoon dried rosemary

¼ teaspoon salt

Freshly ground black pepper (optional)

1 pound pork tenderloin

4 sprigs fresh rosemary (optional)

TIP: You can make this gluten-free by swapping out the panko for almond meal/flour or another crushed nut, rice flour, or ground-up gluten-free cereal like plain Cheerios, Rice Chex, or Corn Chex.

1. Preheat the oven to 375° F. Lightly coat a 9 x 13-inch baking dish with cooking spray.

2. Layer the onion into the baking dish.

3. In a shallow dish, combine the panko, Parmesan, garlic, dried rosemary, salt, and pepper, if desired.

4. Roll the pork tenderloin in the mixture until it is well coated. Place in the baking dish on top of the onion slices.

5. Transfer to the oven and bake, uncovered, until golden and cooked through and an instant-read thermometer reads 145°F, 45 to 50 minutes.

6. Remove from the oven, cover, and allow to rest for 10 minutes before slicing. Garnish with rosemary, if desired.

PER SERVING: Calories: 196; Total fat: 6 g; Saturated fat: 3 g; Cholesterol: 72 mg; Sodium: 316 mg; Potassium: 417 mg; Total carbohydrates: 6 g; Fiber: 1 g; Sugars: <1 g; Protein: 28 g

Restaurant-Style Pork Fajitas

There's no need to go out to eat when you have this quick and healthy recipe for pork fajitas on hand. Just like the restaurant favorite, this recipe uses lean pork tenderloin, colorful and nutrient-rich red and yellow bell peppers, and traditional Tex-Mex flavors topped with avocado slices, fresh cilantro, and fresh lime juice. Incredibly delicious, nutritious, and surprisingly low in calories, this recipe is bound to become a family favorite.

1 tablespoon extra-virgin olive oil

1 pound pork tenderloin, cut into thin strips

1 medium onion, sliced into long strips

1 medium red bell pepper, sliced into long strips

1 medium yellow bell pepper, sliced into long strips

2 cloves garlic, minced

1 teaspoon chili powder

1 teaspoon ground cumin

1 teaspoon smoked paprika

Pinch of cayenne pepper

Salt and freshly ground black pepper (optional)

4 (6-inch) whole-wheat tortillas

1 avocado, sliced

1 lime, cut into wedges

Fresh cilantro

1. In a large skillet, heat ½ tablespoon of the olive oil over medium-high heat until hot. Add the pork and cook until browned and cooked through, 5 to 10 minutes. Remove the pork from the skillet and set aside. Cover to keep warm.

2. Add the remaining ½ tablespoon olive oil to the skillet and heat. Add the onion, bell peppers, and garlic and sprinkle with the chili powder, cumin, smoked paprika, cayenne, and salt and black pepper, if desired. Cook, stirring constantly until the onion is beginning to caramelize and the peppers are softened, 4 to 5 minutes. Return the pork to the skillet, mix with the vegetables and spices, and cook for 1 to 2 minutes to heat through.

3. Meanwhile, wrap the tortillas in paper towels and microwave on high for 3 minutes to warm.

4. To serve, portion the pork and vegetable mixture into the tortillas, and top with avocado slices, a squeeze of fresh lime juice, and fresh cilantro.

PER SERVING: Calories: 366; Total fat: 16 g; Saturated fat: 3 g; Cholesterol: 67 mg; Sodium: 203 mg; Potassium: 774 mg; Total carbohydrates: 29 g; Fiber: 8 g; Sugars: 2 g; Protein: 29 g

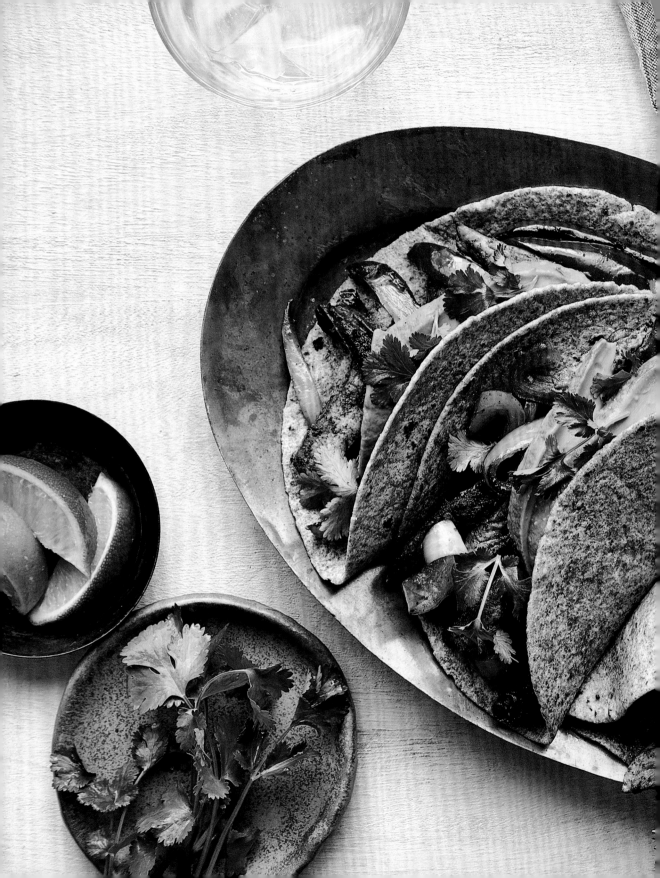

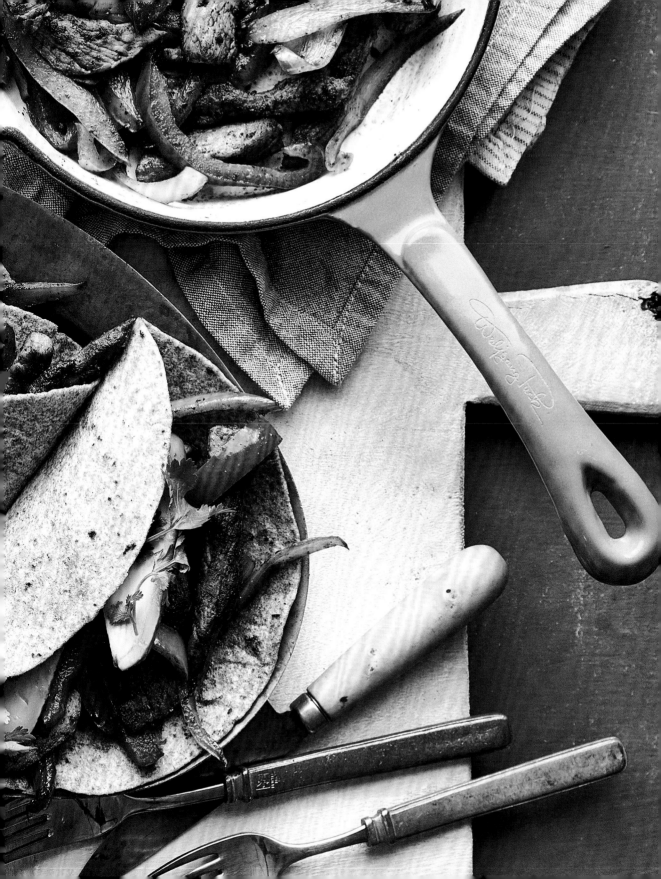

Easy Skillet Swiss Steak

Swiss steak is a common dish in the area of the country where I grew up (Pennsylvania Dutch country), and it is traditionally slow-cooked in the oven for an hour or more, or cooked in a slow cooker. This recipe is adapted from a version one of my aunts used to make, and cuts down on the cook time by cooking the meat in a skillet on the stovetop. The use of cube steak keeps this recipe lean and healthy, and the ample amounts of tomatoes, peppers, and onion ensure you get several servings of nutrient- and fiber-rich vegetables in each portion. Feel free to put your own personal spin on this family favorite.

4 cube steaks (4 ounces each)

¼ teaspoon salt

½ teaspoon freshly ground black pepper

¼ cup whole-wheat or all-purpose flour

2 tablespoons extra-virgin olive oil

1 large onion, sliced

2 medium carrots, sliced into very thin rounds

2 celery stalks, diced

1 medium green bell pepper, chopped

1 medium red or yellow bell pepper, chopped

1 teaspoon sweet paprika

1 (14-ounce) can no-salt-added stewed tomatoes

1 tablespoon Worcestershire sauce

1 orange, peeled and sliced

1. Sprinkle the steaks with the salt and pepper. Place the flour in a shallow dish and dredge the steaks in it.

2. In a large skillet, heat 1 tablespoon of the olive oil over medium-high heat. Reduce the heat to medium, add the steaks, and cook until browned on one side, 3 to 4 minutes. Flip and continue cooking until the other side is browned, 3 to 4 minutes. Transfer to a plate and cover with foil to keep warm.

3. Heat the remaining 1 tablespoon olive oil in the skillet over medium-high heat. Add the onion slices and cook until starting to brown, 4 to 5 minutes. Add the carrots, celery, and bell peppers and cook until the vegetables are tender, stirring occasionally, 6 to 8 minutes.

4. Stir in the paprika, stewed tomatoes and their juices, and Worcestershire sauce and cook, stirring until the sauce thickens, 4 to 5 minutes.

5. Push the vegetables to the sides of the pan and return the steaks to the pan. Layer each steak with the orange slices, simmering for 1 minute, until warmed.

6. To serve, portion the vegetables onto 4 serving plates and top each serving with a steak and the orange slices.

PER SERVING: Calories: 345; Total fat: 16 g; Saturated fat: 6 g; Cholesterol: 62 mg; Sodium: 321 mg; Potassium: 651 mg; Total carbohydrates: 25 g; Fiber: 6 g; Sugars: 11 g; Protein: 29 g

Steak with Red Onions, Peppers, and Mushrooms

This simple and quick steak-and-veggie recipe uses lean top round steak (which is very low in unhealthy fats), and the generous portions of onion, peppers, and mushrooms ensure that half of your plate is filled with fiber-rich veggies. The vegetable mix is the perfect complement to the steak, adding lots of juicy flavor and health-promoting vitamins and minerals without the use of significant amounts of added fat. Serve this meal with brown rice and a fresh salad of baby greens.

- 8 ounces top round steak
- Salt and freshly ground black pepper
- 4 teaspoons extra-virgin olive oil
- 2 cloves garlic, minced
- ½ medium red onion, sliced into rings
- 1 small red bell pepper, sliced into big chunks
- 1 small green bell pepper, sliced into big chunks
- 1 cup sliced baby bella mushrooms

TIP: Mushrooms are an inexpensive, low-calorie, fiber- and nutrient-rich vegetable, and are a delicious complement to any cuisine, adding volume, which can fill you up on less calories. Earthy and meaty tasting, this little veggie is a good source of the antioxidant selenium and the heart-healthy mineral potassium.

1. Slice the beef into thin strips. Season with a dash each of salt and black pepper.

2. Heat a large skillet over high heat. When the skillet is hot, add 1 teaspoon of the olive oil and half of the beef. Cook 1 minute, then flip the steak strips and cook an additional 30 seconds. Set aside in a large dish.

3. Add another 1 teaspoon olive oil to the skillet and heat over high heat. Add the remaining steak, cook 1 minute, then flip and cook an additional 30 seconds. Set aside with the other cooked steak.

4. Add another 1 teaspoon olive oil to the skillet over high heat. Add the garlic, onion, and bell peppers and cook until the onion is golden and the peppers are soft, 3 to 4 minutes. Add the cooked vegetables to the dish with the steak.

5. Reduce the heat under the skillet to medium, add the remaining 1 teaspoon olive oil and the mushrooms and cook for 2 minutes. Return the steak and cooked vegetables to the skillet with the mushrooms, stir to combine, and cook for 1 minute, just to heat through.

6. Serve hot.

PER SERVING: Calories: 293; Total fat: 14 g; Saturated fat: 3 g; Cholesterol: 75 mg; Sodium: 76 mg; Potassium: 224 mg; Total carbohydrates: 12 g; Fiber: 2 g; Sugars: 5 g; Protein: 28 g

Open-Faced Veggie-Packed Beef Burger

The DASH diet recommends that red meat be eaten in moderation. Choose lean cuts and use healthy cooking techniques when preparing red meat. This recipe is a delicious and healthy combination of lean ground beef, cooked beans, and moist veggies for the ultimate veggie-packed beef burger. Quick to prepare and perfect for the grill, this burger should satisfy even diehard beef fans. The veggies allow you to use less meat, add valuable nutrients and fiber, and, with a bit of calcium-rich cheese, keep the burger nice and juicy. Feel free to use your favorite veggies or swap out a veggie for a shredded apple. A combination of healthy and hearty, serve these burgers with a side of roasted sweet potato fries.

½ cup cooked pinto beans (or other bean)

½ cup minced onion

½ cup minced mushrooms

½ cup finely chopped red bell pepper

1 medium carrot, grated

1 medium zucchini, grated

2 cloves garlic, minced

¾ pound 94% lean ground beef (grass-fed if possible; see Tip)

1 tablespoon ground mustard

½ cup shredded low-fat cheddar cheese

Salt and freshly ground black pepper

1 tablespoon extra-virgin olive oil

Lettuce leaves or whole-wheat buns

Optional toppings: avocado slices, tomato slices, fresh parsley

1. In a large bowl, gently mash the beans with the back of a large spoon. Add the onion, mushrooms, bell pepper, carrot, zucchini, garlic, beef, mustard, cheddar, and a dash each of salt and pepper and combine well. Form into 4 patties.

2. In a large skillet, heat the olive oil over medium-high heat. Add the patties and sear them until dark brown on one side, about 5 minutes. Flip and cook for another 5 minutes or until your desired doneness.

3. Serve the burgers on lettuce leaves or toasted buns. Garnish with optional toppings, if desired.

TIP: Beef is one of the biggest sources of saturated fat in the American diet, but it is also an important source of protein, iron, zinc, selenium, and vitamin B_{12}. Luckily, meats like ground beef are sold in different lean-to-fat ratios. According to the USDA, to be labeled "lean" the lean-to-fat ratio must be 92:8 (92% lean, 8% fat) or higher, and for "extra-lean" the ratio must be 96:4 (96% lean, 4% fat).

PER SERVING (WITHOUT BUN OR TOPPINGS): Calories: 226; Total fat: 9 g; Saturated fat: 2 g; Cholesterol: 54 mg; Sodium: 140 mg; Potassium: 390 mg; Total carbohydrates: 12 g; Fiber: 4 g; Sugars: 3 g; Protein: 24 g

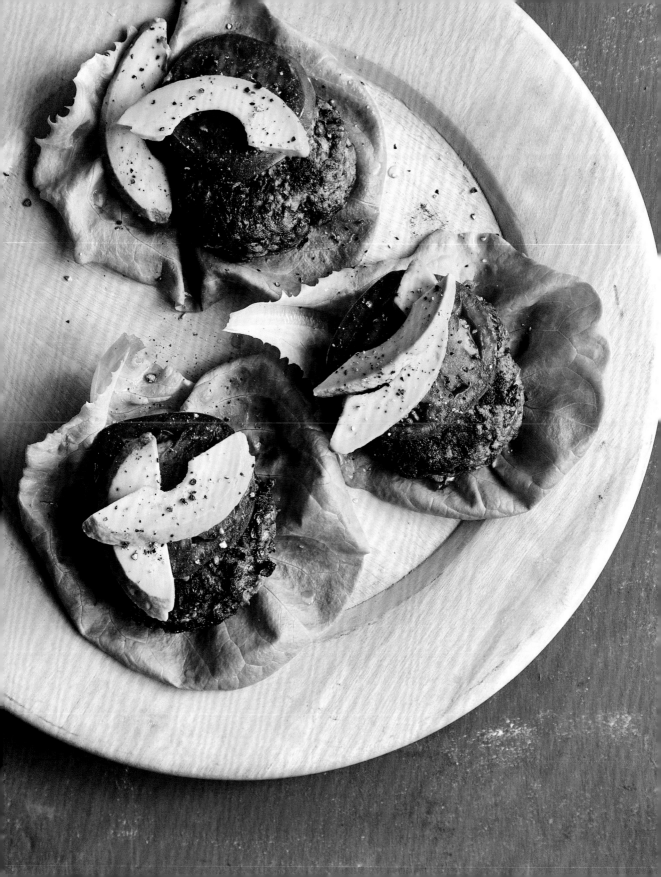

PREP TIME: 10 MINUTES • COOK TIME: 15 MINUTES • SERVES 4

Beef Tenderloin with Chickpeas and Artichoke Hearts

Beef tenderloin is the leanest and most tender cut of beef you can select, and a boneless 4-ounce portion trimmed of fat has just under 160 calories and 6 grams of fat, making it a good choice to include in your DASH weight-loss diet. This recipe cooks the tenderloin quickly in a bit of oil to preserve its tenderness and combines it with the nutritional powerhouses spinach, chickpeas, and artichoke hearts for added antioxidants, vitamins, plant protein, fiber, and blood-pressure-lowering potassium. Seasoned with aromatic sweet-tasting dried marjoram and fresh basil, this nutritious and filling dish is bursting with delicious flavors.

1 tablespoon extra-virgin olive oil

4 beef tenderloin filets (4 ounces each), trimmed of fat

4 cloves garlic, chopped

Pinch of red pepper flakes

4 cups baby spinach

1 (15-ounce) can chickpeas, rinsed and drained

1 (14-ounce) can water-packed artichoke hearts, drained and rinsed

1 cup chopped fresh tomatoes, with their juices

2 teaspoons dried marjoram

1/2 cup chopped fresh basil leaves

Salt and freshly ground black pepper (optional)

1. In a large sauté pan, heat the olive oil over medium-high heat until shimmering. Add the beef and cook until the filets are well browned on the bottom, about 2 minutes. Flip and cook until well browned on the second side, another 2 minutes. Transfer to a plate and cover to keep warm.

2. Reduce the heat under the skillet to medium. Add the garlic and sauté until golden brown, about 1 minute. Add the pepper flakes and spinach. Cook and stir for 1 minute to wilt the spinach. Add 1/2 cup water, then cover the pan and bring to a simmer. Uncover and cook until almost all of the water is evaporated, 3 to 4 minutes.

3. Add the chickpeas, artichoke hearts, tomatoes with their juices, and the marjoram. Cook for 2 minutes and stir to allow the sauce to coat the vegetables.

4. Return the beef to the pan along with any collected juices on the plate and toss in the fresh basil. Cover and cook until the beef is cooked to your desired doneness, 2 to 3 minutes.

5. Place a beef filet on each of 4 serving plates. Season the vegetables with salt and pepper, if desired, and portion onto the plates with the beef.

PER SERVING: Calories: 348; Total fat: 11 g; Saturated fat: 3 g; Cholesterol: 60 mg; Sodium: 129 mg; Potassium: 1,054 mg; Total carbohydrates: 29 g; Fiber: 12 g; Sugars: 4 g; Protein: 34 g

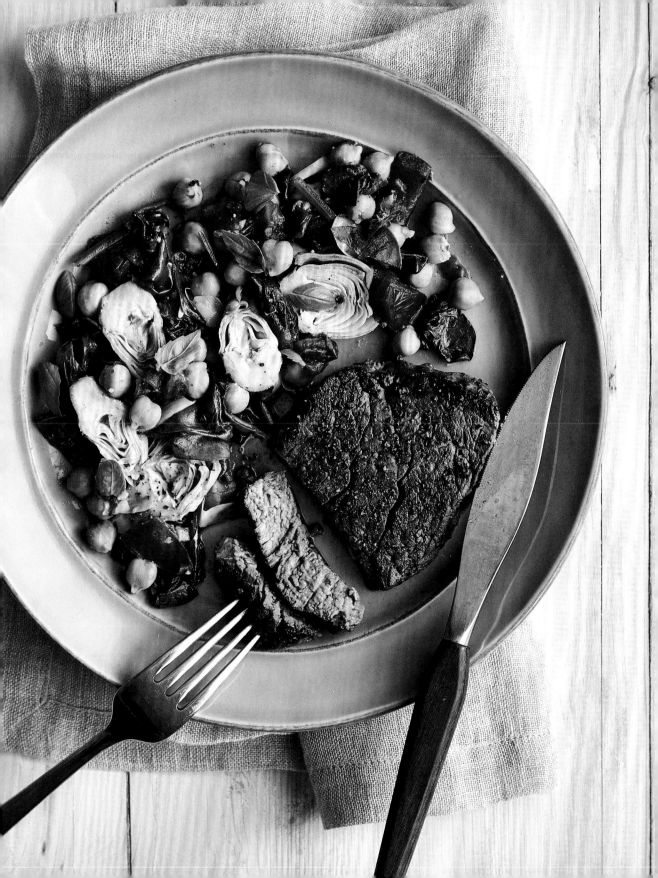

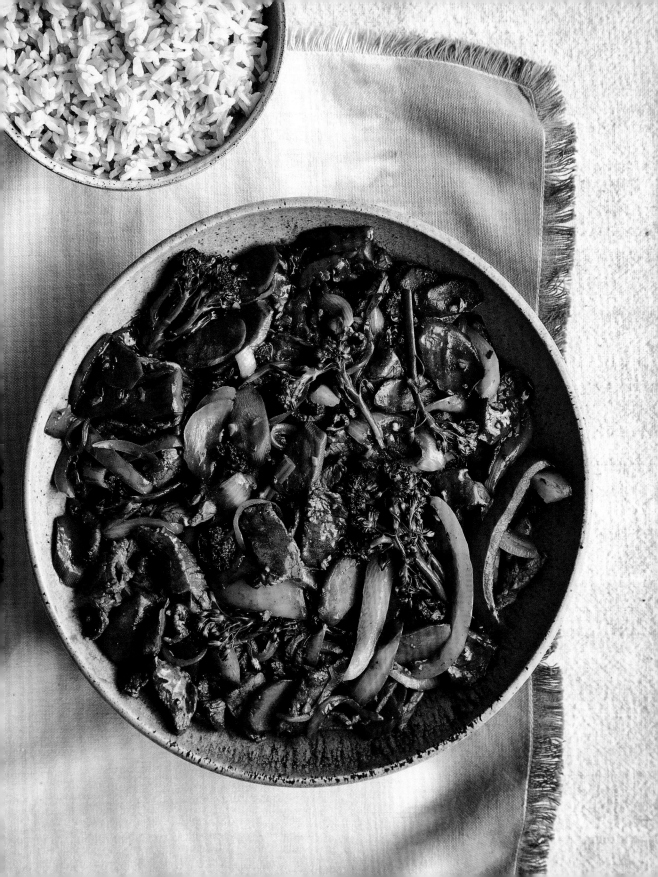

Spicy Sichuan Orange Beef Vegetable Stir-Fry

With all of the traditional flavors of your favorite take-out food but with far less sodium and unhealthy fats, this recipe is perfect when you need to put dinner on the table super fast. Once you make this recipe a few times and find out how quick and easy it is for you to make a delicious spicy beef stir-fry that rivals your restaurant favorite, you just might toss those take-out menus. Serve over hot rice or Herbed Cauliflower and Broccoli Rice (page 211).

¾ cup orange juice

1 tablespoon reduced-sodium soy sauce (see Tip)

1 tablespoon unseasoned rice vinegar or dry sherry

1 teaspoon sesame oil

2 teaspoons cornstarch

¼ teaspoon Chinese five-spice powder

1 teaspoon red pepper flakes

2 teaspoons extra-virgin olive oil

8 ounces boneless beef sirloin steak, cut into thin strips

3 cloves garlic, minced

2 teaspoons grated fresh ginger

3 cups frozen stir-fry vegetable blend

TIP: One thing to remember when watching your sodium intake is that it's your total intake for the whole day that counts. So if you have one meal that is a tad higher in sodium, simply adjust your other meals and make your choices low-sodium or sodium-free. It's all about balance.

1. In a small bowl, combine the orange juice, soy sauce, rice vinegar, sesame oil, cornstarch, five-spice, and pepper flakes until smooth. Set aside.

2. In a large skillet or wok, heat 1 teaspoon of the olive oil over high heat. Add the beef and stir-fry until no longer pink, 3 to 4 minutes. Remove with a slotted spoon to a plate; cover to keep warm.

3. Add the remaining 1 teaspoon olive oil to the pan. Add the garlic and ginger and stir-fry for 1 minute. Add the vegetables and continue cooking for 2 to 3 minutes, until thawed. Stir the sauce and pour into the pan, bring to a boil, and cook for 2 to 3 minutes to thicken. Return the beef to the pan, stir to combine, and cook for an additional 1 to 2 minutes to heat through.

PER SERVING (WITHOUT RICE): Calories: 321; Total fat: 12 g; Saturated fat: 3 g; Cholesterol: 65 mg; Sodium: 376 mg; Potassium: 454 mg; Total carbohydrates: 22 g; Fiber: 4 g; Sugars: 13 g; Protein: 28 g

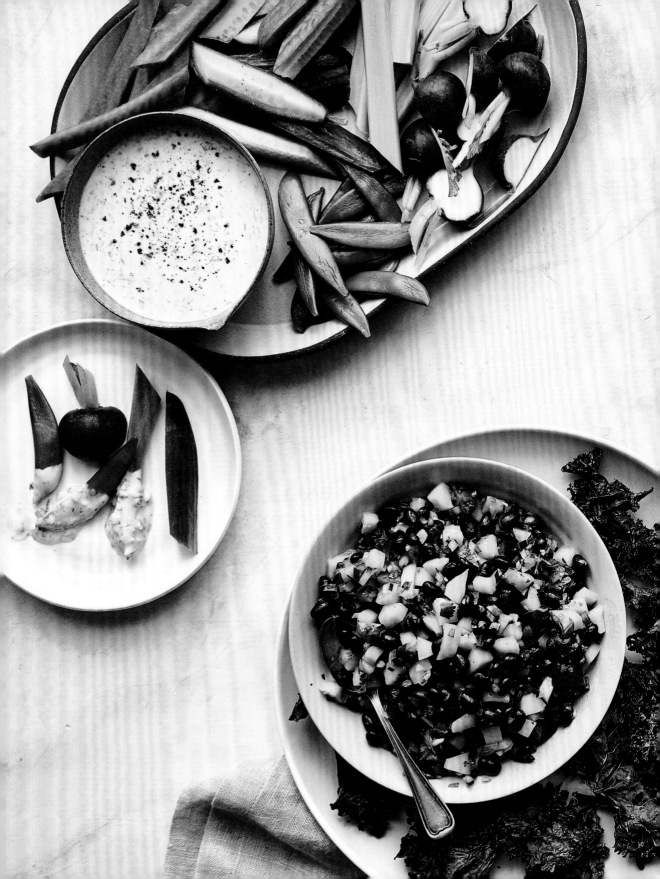

Sauces, Stocks, and Condiments

Roasted Red Pepper and Tomato Sauce

The prep involved in this recipe is well worth it in terms of taste. Intense in flavor, this creamy red sauce is made using red peppers that are roasted and then sautéed and processed with tomato puree. The resulting sauce is packed with flavor and health-promoting antioxidants, vitamins, and minerals. The star of your next pasta dish, this delicious sauce also works well on grains, vegetables, baked potatoes, and grilled meat, fish, and tofu.

3 large red bell peppers (see Tip)

2 tablespoons extra-virgin olive oil, plus more for brushing peppers

1 medium onion, minced

3 cloves garlic, minced

2 teaspoons dried basil

1 teaspoon dried oregano

½ teaspoon dried rosemary

½ cup low-sodium vegetable broth

½ cup no-salt-added tomato sauce

2 tablespoons tomato paste

2 teaspoons white wine vinegar

½ teaspoon salt

2 tablespoons chopped fresh basil

TIP: You can use a combination of sweet bell peppers in this recipe including red, orange, and yellow. Green peppers are not recommended.

1. Preheat the broiler.

2. Cut the bell peppers in half lengthwise, remove the seeds, and press open to flatten. Place the peppers skin side up under the broiler and cook until lightly charred, about 10 minutes. Remove the pepper halves, stacking one on top of the other inside of a small paper bag to create steam or place in a bowl and cover. Let sit 10 minutes, then remove as much charred skin as possible. Slice into strips.

3. In a large skillet, heat the 2 tablespoons olive oil over medium-high heat. Add the pepper strips, onion, garlic, dried basil, oregano, and rosemary and cook, stirring, until the peppers, onion, and garlic have softened and the herbs are fragrant, about 5 minutes.

4. Reduce the heat to medium, add the vegetable broth and cook until the mixture is reduced to a sauce, about 15 minutes.

5. Add the tomato sauce, tomato paste, and 1½ cups water, reduce the heat, and simmer, uncovered, for 25 minutes.

6. Transfer the sauce to a food processor and puree until smooth. Return the sauce to the skillet and bring to a very low simmer. Stir in the vinegar, salt, and basil. Serve warm.

PER ½ CUP: Calories: 92; Total fat: 5 g; Saturated fat: <1 g; Cholesterol: 0 mg; Sodium: 238 mg; Potassium: 364 mg; Total carbohydrates: 11 g; Fiber: 3 g; Sugars: 5 g; Protein: 1 g

Creamy Spinach-Artichoke Sauce

Spinach artichoke dip served in a bread bowl is a popular appetizer that's hard to resist, but one that is high in calories and unhealthy fats because it's made with sour cream, mayonnaise, cream cheese, and Parmesan. This lightened-up DASH version leaves out the mayo and makes some healthy swaps so you can enjoy it as a sauce over grilled chicken or fish or whole-grain pasta—without the chips and without the guilt.

2 teaspoons extra-virgin olive oil

4 cloves garlic, minced

1/2 cup diced onion

1 tablespoon whole-wheat or all-purpose flour

1 cup fat-free milk

1/2 cup shredded part-skim mozzarella cheese (2 ounces)

1/2 cup nonfat (0%) plain Greek yogurt

2 ounces 1/3-less-fat cream cheese

10 ounces frozen chopped spinach, thawed and squeezed of excess water (see Tip)

1 (14-ounce) can water-packed artichoke hearts, rinsed, drained, and chopped

1/4 cup grated Parmesan cheese

1/4 teaspoon salt

1/2 teaspoon freshly ground black pepper

1/2 teaspoon red pepper flakes

1/4 teaspoon grated lemon zest

1. In a large skillet, heat the olive oil over medium heat. Add the garlic and onion and cook until softened, 3 to 4 minutes. Add the flour and stir until the flour begins to brown. Stir in the milk and bring to a boil, then immediately reduce the heat to low and simmer for 3 to 4 minutes, until it starts to thicken.

2. Add the mozzarella, Greek yogurt, and cream cheese and stir until melted, 2 to 3 minutes. Add the spinach and artichoke hearts and cook stirring constantly for 3 to 4 minutes to warm through.

3. Add the Parmesan, salt, black pepper, pepper flakes, and lemon zest and cook until the cheese has melted and the ingredients are thoroughly combined, an additional 2 to 3 minutes.

4. Serve immediately or refrigerate in a covered container for 3 to 4 days.

TIP: It's important to squeeze out the excess water from the frozen spinach so that it doesn't make the sauce watery. An easy way to do this is to line a colander with either a kitchen towel or paper towels, then place the thawed spinach on the towels and wrap them around the spinach, squeezing out the excess water. Doing it over the colander ensures you don't lose your spinach if the paper towels break.

PER 1/3 CUP: Calories: 104; Total fat: 4 g; Saturated fat: 2 g; Cholesterol: 9 mg; Sodium: 244 mg; Potassium: 394 mg; Total carbohydrates: 11 g; Fiber: 5 g; Sugars: 3 g; Protein: 8 g

Black Bean Mango Salsa

There's nothing better than freshly prepared salsa, and this recipe can check off a number of boxes for you on your DASH eating plan. With protein, fiber, vitamins, and minerals from black beans, and vitamin C from sweet mango, you can whip up this flavorful, fiery salsa in minutes. With a balance of sweet and spicy, this salsa tastes terrific served over homemade burritos or tofu scramble, spooned over grilled fish or chicken, or served with Cheesy Baked Kale Chips (page 209).

1 large mango, finely diced

1 (15-ounce) can black beans, rinsed and drained

¼ cup finely minced red onion

2 cloves garlic, minced

1 Roma (plum) tomato (see Tip), coarsely chopped

½ to 1 jalapeño pepper, seeded and diced

½ cup chopped fresh cilantro

Juice of 1 lime

Pinch of salt

1. In a medium bowl, combine the mango, black beans, onion, garlic, tomato, jalapeño to taste, the cilantro, lime juice, and salt and stir to combine. Cover and refrigerate for at least 10 minutes and up to one day to meld the flavors.

2. Store in an airtight container in the refrigerator for 5 to 7 days.

3. Taste the salsa before serving and adjust seasonings to taste.

PER 2 TABLESPOONS: Calories: 17; Total fat: 0 g; Saturated fat: 0 g; Cholesterol: 0 mg; Sodium: 3 mg; Potassium: 21 mg; Total carbohydrates: 3 g; Fiber: 1 g; Sugars: 1 g; Protein: 1 g

TIP: Roma tomatoes are a good choice for salsa because they contain few seeds and have a meaty interior full of flavor.

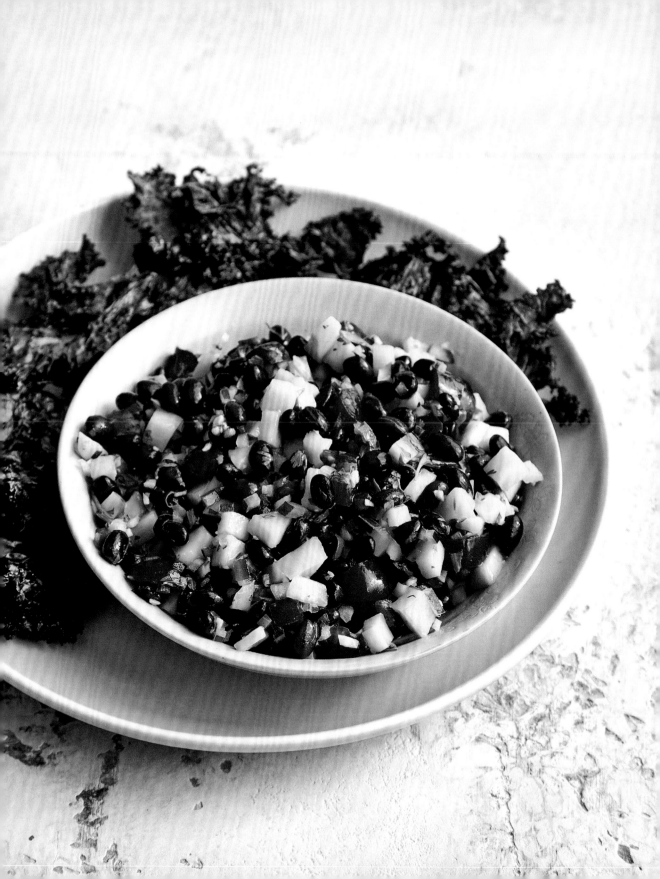

Fresh Cranberry Sauce

Cranberries don't always get the attention they deserve in terms of their health benefits; however, they more than earn their place among phytonutrient-rich foods. Extremely high in antioxidants and anti-inflammatory compounds, cranberries can help keep cholesterol in check and promote a healthy blood pressure. Available in most grocery stores year-round fresh and frozen, use them to prepare this four-ingredient homemade cranberry sauce that is ready in less than 10 minutes. Use as a topping for grilled fish or chicken or spoon over Greek yogurt or cooked oats.

2 cups fresh or frozen cranberries

Juice of 1 orange

1 teaspoon grated fresh ginger

¼ cup granulated no-calorie sweetener (e.g., stevia)

TIP: Along with making a healthy side for your Thanksgiving turkey, this sauce tastes delicious on sweet potatoes, veggie or meat burgers, as a replacement for high-sugar jam on toast, as an add-in to tuna salad, or as a stuffing for baked acorn squash.

1. In a medium saucepan, combine the cranberries, ¾ cup water, the orange juice, ginger, and sweetener. Bring to a boil while stirring constantly and cook until the cranberries burst, about 5 minutes.

2. Transfer to a food processor or blender and process gently for 30 seconds.

3. Serve warm or store in an airtight container in the refrigerator for up to 2 weeks. You can also freeze the sauce in freezer bags.

PER ¼ CUP: Calories: 29; Total fat: <1 g; Saturated fat: 0 g; Cholesterol: 0 mg; Sodium: 1 mg; Potassium: 74 mg; Total carbohydrates: 8 g; Fiber: 2 g; Sugars: 3 g; Protein: <1 g

Asian Ginger Stir-Fry Sauce

Skip the processed, high-calorie, overly salty stir-fry sauces and make your own in minutes. With intense Asian flavor from soy, ginger, garlic, sesame oil, and rice vinegar, this sauce can be used with any combination of vegetables and type of meat including beef, shrimp, chicken, and pork, and with plant-based stir-fries using tofu. Store this in the refrigerator and when using in your stir-fries, allow the sauce to cook for 3 to 4 minutes in order for the cornstarch to thicken.

¼ cup reduced-sodium soy sauce (or tamari for gluten-free)

¼ cup low-sodium vegetable broth

1 teaspoon cornstarch, plus more as needed

1 teaspoon honey

Juice of 1 lime

1 teaspoon sesame oil

1 teaspoon rice vinegar

2 cloves garlic, minced

1 tablespoon grated fresh ginger (see Tip)

Dash of hot chili sauce (optional)

In a small bowl, whisk together the soy sauce, vegetable broth, cornstarch, honey, lime juice, sesame oil, rice vinegar, garlic, ginger, and chili sauce (if using). (The sauce will thicken up quickly with 1 teaspoon of cornstarch, but if necessary, add 1 additional teaspoon to achieve your preferred consistency). Refrigerate in an airtight container for up to 7 days. Before using, whisk to incorporate the cornstarch.

PER 2 TABLESPOONS: Calories: 32; Total fat: <1 g; Saturated fat: <1 g; Cholesterol: 0 mg; Sodium: 448 mg; Potassium: 26 mg; Total carbohydrates: 4 g; Fiber: <1 g; Sugars: 3 g; Protein: <1 g

TIP: Ginger is available in most grocery stores as a paste sold in a tube in the produce aisle with the other herbs. This is a nice option because it lasts much longer than the root, and also cuts down on prep time.

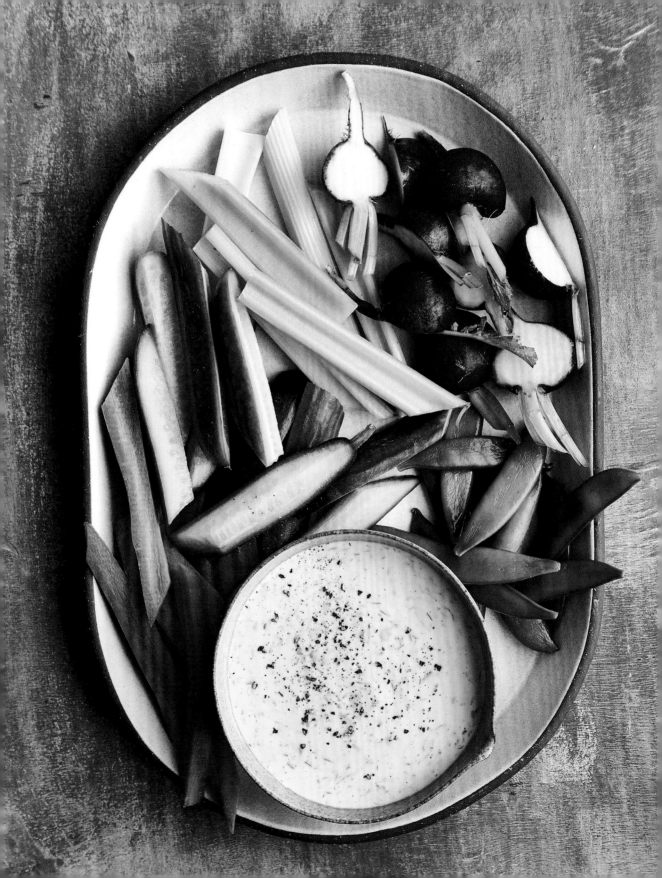

PREP TIME: 5 MINUTES • MAKES 2 CUPS

Herbed Greek Yogurt Dressing

This delicious calcium- and protein-rich dressing takes just minutes to prepare and is much healthier and lighter than traditional creamy dressings. Use on top of salads, over fresh vegetables, or on top of burgers and burritos. Easy, creamy, and delicious, add your favorite fresh herbs.

¼ cup chopped fresh dill

¼ cup chopped chives

½ cup chopped fresh parsley

1 small shallot, minced

2 cloves garlic, chopped

1 cup nonfat (0%) plain Greek yogurt

2 tablespoons extra-virgin olive oil

2 tablespoons juice from 1 lemon

½ teaspoon honey

⅛ teaspoon salt

⅛ teaspoon freshly ground black pepper

1. In a food processor, combine the dill, chives, and parsley and pulse a few times until they have been ground up slightly. Scrape down the sides.

2. Add the shallot, garlic, Greek yogurt, olive oil, lemon juice, ¼ cup water (see Tips), the honey, salt, and pepper and pulse until smooth and the ingredients have been fully incorporated.

3. Use immediately or store in an airtight container in the refrigerator for up to 1 week.

PER 2 TABLESPOONS: Calories: 26; Total fat: 2 g; Saturated fat: <1 g; Cholesterol: <1 mg; Sodium: 27 mg; Potassium: 53 mg; Total carbohydrates: 1 g; Fiber: <1 g; Sugars: 1 g; Protein: 2 g

TIPS: Although meant to be prepared with fresh herbs, dried can substitute in a pinch. One teaspoon dried is roughly equivalent to 1 tablespoon fresh.

You can also easily turn this dressing into a dip by eliminating the water.

Vegetable Broth

Making your own vegetable broth is easy to do and can help cut down on food waste while being a much healthier alternative to high-sodium processed varieties. You can use this recipe as a guide and substitute the 5 or 6 cups of the vegetable trimmings you have on hand. Once finished, use the broth in place of water to enhance the flavor of rice and other cooked grains or as a base for homemade soups and gravies.

1 medium potato, chopped into large chunks

1 onion, quartered

2 celery stalks, chopped

2 carrots, chopped

6 cloves garlic, smashed

8 whole black peppercorns

2 bay leaves

2 teaspoons dried thyme

TIP: You can also make this in a slow cooker and cook on LOW for 8 to 12 hours. The longer it cooks, the more flavor and nutrients are extracted from the ingredients.

1. In a large soup pot or Dutch oven (see Tip), combine the potato, onion, celery, carrots, garlic, peppercorns, bay leaves, thyme, and 7 cups water. Bring to a boil, then reduce the heat to low, cover, and let simmer for at least 1 hour.

2. Strain the broth (discard the solids) and refrigerate in an airtight container for up to 5 days or freeze in 1-cup portions.

PER 1 CUP: Calories: 29; Total fat: <1 g; Saturated fat: 0 g; Cholesterol: 0 mg; Sodium: 16 mg; Potassium: 0 mg; Total carbohydrates: 6 g; Fiber: <1 g; Sugars: <1 g; Protein: <1 g

Raspberry-Tarragon Vinaigrette

This sweet and delicious raspberry-tarragon vinaigrette is quick to prepare and tastes wonderful on a fresh green salad, or as a topping for steamed vegetables or cooked grains. High in antioxidants with healthy fats from olive oil, use this nutrient-dense homemade version in place of store-bought varieties that often contain too much salt, sugar, and preservatives.

½ cup fresh raspberries (do not use frozen; see Tip)

2 tablespoons white wine vinegar

1 clove garlic, minced

1 tablespoon minced shallot

1 teaspoon honey

⅛ teaspoon salt

2 tablespoons extra-virgin olive oil

1 teaspoon dried tarragon

1. In a blender or food processor, puree the raspberries, vinegar, garlic, shallot, honey, and salt. Pour into a small bowl.

2. Add the olive oil in a thin stream while whisking constantly. Stir in the tarragon.

3. Use immediately or store in an airtight container in the refrigerator for up to 2 days.

PER 2 TABLESPOONS: Calories: 48; Total fat: 4 g; Saturated fat: <1 g; Cholesterol: 0 mg; Sodium: 73 mg; Potassium: 48 mg; Total carbohydrates: 4 g; Fiber: 1 g; Sugars: 2 g; Protein: <1 g

TIP: You can swap out the raspberries for blueberries or strawberries. Add a teaspoon of poppy seeds for another healthy twist on this dressing.

Red Lentil and Roasted Walnut Spread

This delicious and creamy pâté-like spread—which combines the health benefits of two DASH-recommended foods, lentils and walnuts, to create a spread rich in protein, fiber, and omega-3 fatty acids—is sure to please everyone. A nice change of pace from hummus, use this as a sandwich spread, a dip for vegetables, or as a topping for whole-grain pasta. This spread is naturally vegan and gluten-free.

1 cup red lentils, rinsed (see Tip)

½ cup walnuts, chopped

1 shallot, chopped

2 cloves garlic, chopped

1 teaspoon dried thyme

½ teaspoon sweet paprika

2 tablespoons tomato paste

2 teaspoons fresh lemon juice

¼ teaspoon salt

¼ teaspoon freshly ground black pepper

TIP: I like using the smaller split red lentils in this recipe because they tend to disintegrate when cooked, and work well in recipes where they are pureed. However, it's perfectly fine to use brown or green lentils—just note that the cooking time will be about 5 to 10 minutes longer.

1. In a small saucepan, combine the lentils and 2 cups water and bring to a boil over high heat. Reduce the heat to low, cover, and simmer until the lentils are tender but not mushy and the water is absorbed, about 15 minutes. Drain well. Transfer to a food processor.

2. Meanwhile, in a dry medium skillet, toast the walnuts over low heat, stirring constantly, until they start to brown and are fragrant, 2 to 3 minutes. Scrape them into the food processor over the lentils.

3. Add the shallot, garlic, thyme, paprika, tomato paste, lemon juice, salt, and pepper to the food processor. Process the mixture until smooth and well combined, stopping occasionally to scrape the bowl down. If the mixture is too thick, add water 1 tablespoon at a time until you achieve a smooth spreadable consistency similar to hummus.

4. Serve immediately or store in an airtight container in the refrigerator for up to 5 days.

PER ¼ CUP: Calories: 70; Total fat: 2 g; Saturated fat: <1 g; Cholesterol: 0 mg; Sodium: 38 mg; Potassium: 49 mg; Total carbohydrates: 8 g; Fiber: 1 g; Sugars: 1 g; Protein: 4 g

Protein-Packed Guacamole

There's no need to feel deprived of your favorites when you are managing your weight and eating to improve your health. The secret to this guacamole recipe is the addition of protein- and fiber-rich green peas. Peas sounds like an odd thing to put in guacamole, but they add a thicker texture and slight sweetness to the dip, while simultaneously boosting the protein content and reducing the fat and calories. Protein is the nutrient that keeps us full the longest, so it's a delicious win-win. Just toss everything into a food processor and enjoy with your favorite veggie sticks or Mexican dishes.

3 small avocados, halved and pitted

1 cup frozen green peas, thawed (see Tip)

3 cloves garlic, minced

¼ cup fresh lime juice

½ teaspoon freshly ground black pepper

¼ teaspoon salt

1 medium tomato, chopped

1 jalapeño pepper, seeded and chopped

½ cup finely chopped fresh cilantro

1. Scrape the avocado flesh out of the skins and into a food processor or a high-powered blender. Add the peas, garlic, lime juice, pepper, and salt and pulse to combine. Add the tomato, jalapeño, and cilantro and pulse until smooth.

2. Transfer to a bowl and chill in the refrigerator until ready to serve.

PER ¼ CUP: Calories: 115; Total fat: 8 g; Saturated fat: 1 g; Cholesterol: 0 mg; Sodium: 104 mg; Potassium: 387 mg; Total carbohydrates: 10 g; Fiber: 6 g; Sugars: 2 g; Protein: 3 g

TIP: You can also make this with shelled edamame instead of green peas for an equally creamy, tasty guacamole. Edamame has slightly more protein, calories, and healthy fat than peas, so note that the substitution will change the nutrition calculation of the recipe.

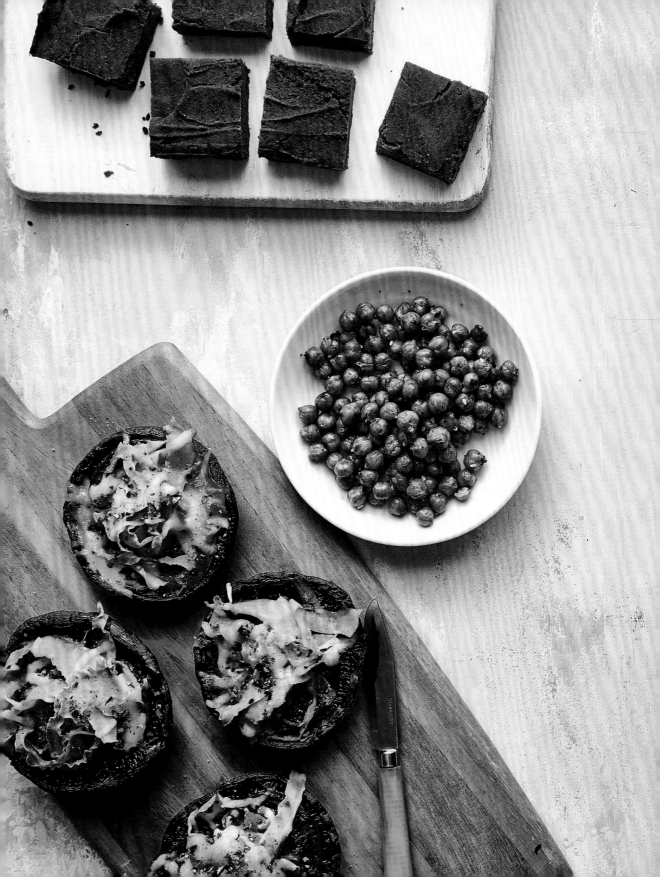

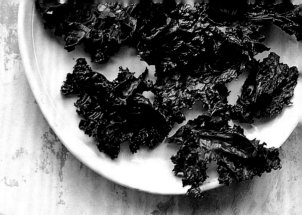

Snacks, Sides, and Desserts

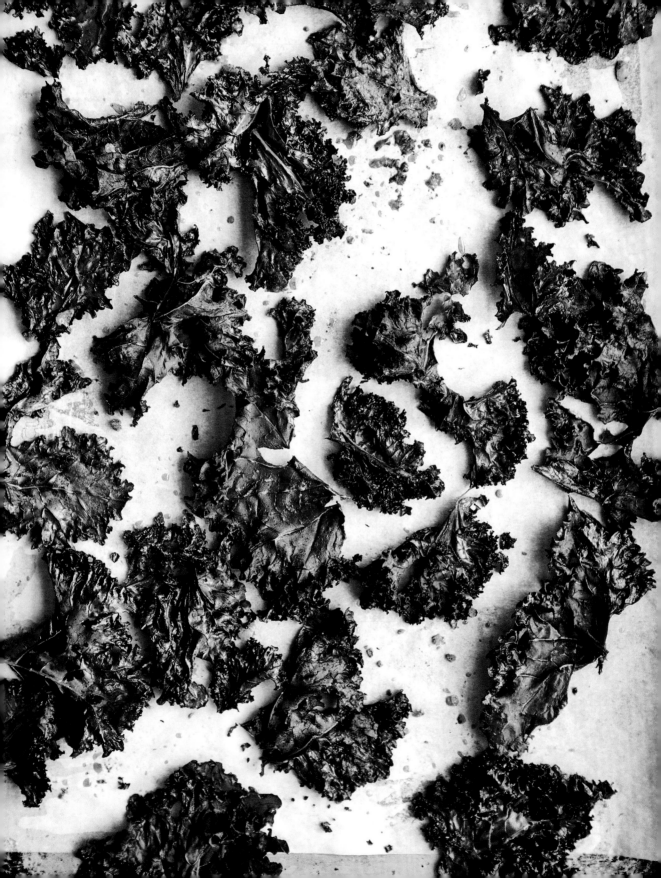

Cheesy Baked Kale Chips

Homemade kale chips are super easy to make and far less pricey than the store-bought variety. Plus, when you make your own, you can control the amount of salt and other seasonings that are added. Because they are homemade, they don't keep long, but that shouldn't be a problem—when you taste how good they are, you'll eat them right up! A healthy alternative to potato chips, enjoy these as a healthy afternoon snack with homemade hummus.

- 1 large bunch curly green or purple kale, stems and midrib removed
- 1 tablespoon avocado oil, olive oil, grapeseed oil, or hazelnut oil
- 2 tablespoons grated Parmesan cheese (or for vegan chips, 2 tablespoons nutritional yeast)
- Pinch of salt
- 1 teaspoon seasoning of choice: such as cumin, curry powder, chili powder, etc.

1. Preheat the oven to 300°F (see Tip). Line 2 large baking sheets with parchment paper.

2. Discard the stem and pull out the tough midrib from the kale leaves. Roughly tear the leaves into large pieces. Wash the leaves and thoroughly dry.

3. Place the leaves in a large bowl and drizzle with the oil. Use your hands to massage the oil into the leaves to soften the texture ensuring all of the nooks and crannies are coated. Next sprinkle with the Parmesan, salt, and seasoning of choice and toss with your hands to combine, working it into the kale to ensure it is thoroughly coated.

4. Spread the kale out evenly into a single layer on the baking sheets, being certain to not overcrowd the kale.

5. Transfer the kale to the oven and bake for 10 minutes, then rotate the baking sheet front to back and continue baking for another 10 to 15 minutes. The kale will shrink as it firms up and get crispy and the edges will begin to brown slightly. You don't want the kale to burn, so be certain to keep an eye on it.

6. Remove the kale from the oven and allow to cool slightly, 3 to 5 minutes, before enjoying. Note that after 24 hours the crispy texture begins to soften, so plan on enjoying the same day. If needed, store the remainder in an airtight container for 2 to 3 days.

TIP: The key to perfect kale chips is baking at a lower temperature, so don't be tempted to speed things along by increasing the temperature, as this will result in burning.

PER SERVING: Calories: 79; Total fat: 5 g; Saturated fat: 1 g; Cholesterol: 2 mg; Sodium: 92 mg; Potassium: 296 mg; Total carbohydrates: 7 g; Fiber: 3 g; Sugars: 2 g; Protein: 3 g

No-Bake Stuffed Mini Peppers

Mini sweet peppers are perfectly stuff-able and make a nutritious snack or game day appetizer. Colorful and full of health-promoting antioxidants, each mini pepper has only about 25 calories and offers heart-healthy potassium, vitamin C, folate, and B vitamins. No baking required, these little veggies are stuffed with a creamy blend of protein- and fiber-rich chickpeas, calcium- and protein-rich ricotta cheese, and delicious herbs and spices.

1 (16-ounce) bag sweet mini peppers (about 16 mini peppers)

1 (15-ounce) can chickpeas, rinsed and drained

½ cup part-skim ricotta cheese (see Tip)

2 teaspoons extra-virgin olive oil

1 teaspoon dried dill

1 teaspoon garlic powder

¼ teaspoon freshly ground black pepper

¼ teaspoon salt

1. Cut the stems off the peppers and halve the peppers lengthwise. Remove any seeds that are inside. Set aside.

2. In a food processor, combine the chickpeas, ricotta, olive oil, dill, garlic powder, black pepper, and salt and pulse 4 or 5 times. The mixture should still have some texture to it.

3. Stuff each pepper half with about 2 tablespoons of the mixture.

4. Serve immediately or store in an airtight container and refrigerate for up to 3 days.

TIP: Make this vegan by replacing the ricotta cheese with nondairy yogurt or silken tofu. For a variation, use a can of rinsed and drained black beans and swap the dill for cumin.

PER SERVING: Calories: 93; Total fat: 3 g; Saturated fat: <1 g; Cholesterol: 5 mg; Sodium: 113 mg; Potassium: 211 mg; Total carbohydrates: 13 g; Fiber: 3 g; Sugars: 4 g; Protein: 5 g

PREP TIME: 5 MINUTES · COOK TIME: 10 MINUTES · SERVES 4

Herbed Cauliflower and Broccoli Rice

Using riced vegetables to create a seasoned side dish in place of a higher-calorie grain or starchy vegetable is a great way to help you to manage your weight. Plus, focusing on filling your plate with high-volume, low-calorie foods is a smart strategy for making meals satisfying and filling so you never have to leave the table feeling hungry. This flavorful recipe is rich in fiber, vitamins, and minerals, and is perfectly seasoned with nutrient-rich leeks, garlic, thyme, and fresh parsley. Olive oil and pine nuts add healthy fats. Feel free to use your favorite herbs and nuts.

1 tablespoon extra-virgin olive oil

1 leek, chopped

3 cloves garlic, minced

2 cups riced cauliflower

2 cups riced broccoli (or use all cauliflower, see Tips)

Pinch of salt

¼ teaspoon freshly ground black pepper

2 teaspoons dried thyme

¼ cup pine nuts

¼ cup chopped fresh parsley

1. In a large skillet, heat the olive oil over medium-high heat. Add the leek and cook until softened, 2 to 3 minutes. Add the garlic and cook for 1 minute, stirring.

2. Add the riced cauliflower and broccoli, season with the salt and pepper, and stir until heated through, 5 to 6 minutes.

3. Remove from the heat and stir in the thyme, pine nuts, and fresh parsley.

PER SERVING: Calories: 133; Total fat: 10 g; Saturated fat: 1 g; Cholesterol: 0 mg; Sodium: 50 mg; Potassium: 393 mg; Total carbohydrates: 10 g; Fiber: 2 g; Sugars: 2 g; Protein: 4 g

TIPS: Riced vegetables are readily available in the fresh produce section and in the frozen vegetable section. You might even mix things up and add a bit of riced sweet potato, beet, or zucchini depending on your preferences.

To use this as a rice substitute for recipes like Almond Butter Tofu and Roasted Asparagus (page 147), simply replace the thyme with ground ginger and omit the pine nuts and parsley.

Snacks, Sides, and Desserts   **211**

Butternut Squash and Sage Portobello Mushroom Pizzas

Portobello mushroom pizzas are a simple, quick, and delicious way to enjoy this beloved dish without any of the guilt. These hearty caps are meaty to the bite, full of fiber and heart-healthy nutrients, and each cap has only about 22 calories. Easy to customize with your favorite toppings, this recipe satisfies pizza cravings while boosting your fiber and veggie intake at the same time. A unique twist on toppings, this recipe uses butternut squash ribbons and fresh sage paired with fresh tomatoes and mozzarella to create a perfectly balanced and healthy snack.

4 large portobello mushroom caps (about 3 ounces each), washed and stems removed (see Tip)

4 teaspoons extra-virgin olive oil

1 Roma (plum) tomato, thinly sliced

1 cup butternut squash ribbons (or spirals)

½ cup shredded part-skim mozzarella cheese (2 ounces)

4 teaspoons minced fresh sage

1 teaspoon red pepper flakes

1 teaspoon garlic powder

Salt and freshly ground black pepper (optional)

1. Preheat the oven to 350°F.

2. Place a wire rack over a rimmed baking sheet and place the mushroom caps gill side up on top of the rack (this keeps the mushrooms from getting soggy).

3. Drizzle each cap with 1 teaspoon olive oil. Layer each cap with 1 or 2 slices tomato, followed by ¼ cup butternut squash ribbons, 2 tablespoons mozzarella cheese, 1 teaspoon fresh sage, ¼ teaspoon pepper flakes, ¼ teaspoon garlic powder, and salt and pepper, if desired.

4. Transfer to the oven and bake until the mushrooms have softened and the cheese has melted, 25 to 30 minutes.

TIP: I like keeping the gills in the mushrooms, but if you prefer, you can gently scoop them out using a spoon. Just be careful not to puncture the cap.

PER SERVING: Calories: 130; Total fat: 7 g; Saturated fat: 2 g; Cholesterol: 7 mg; Sodium: 78 mg; Potassium: 529 mg; Total carbohydrates: 10 g; Fiber: 3 g; Sugars: 0 g; Protein: 8 g

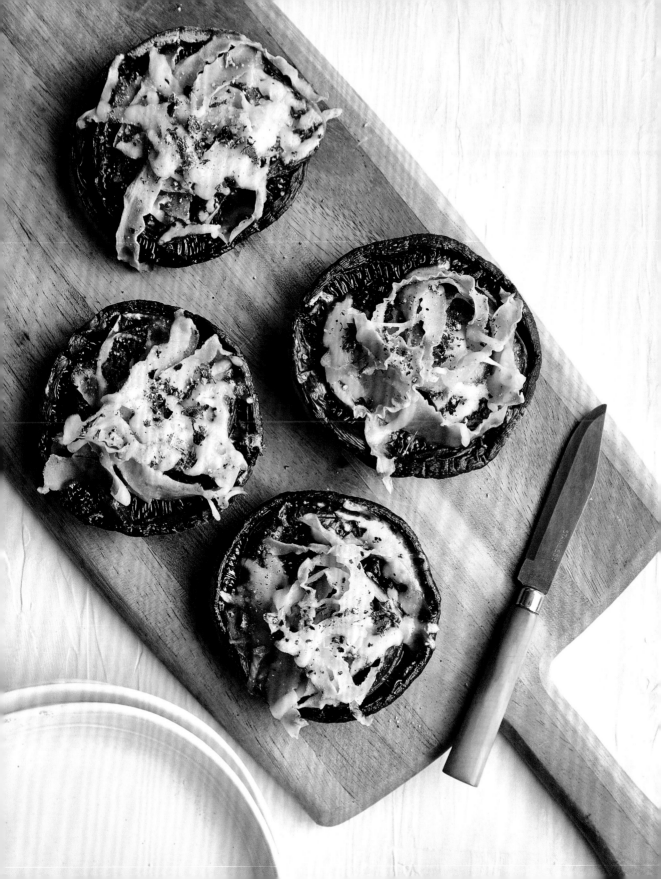

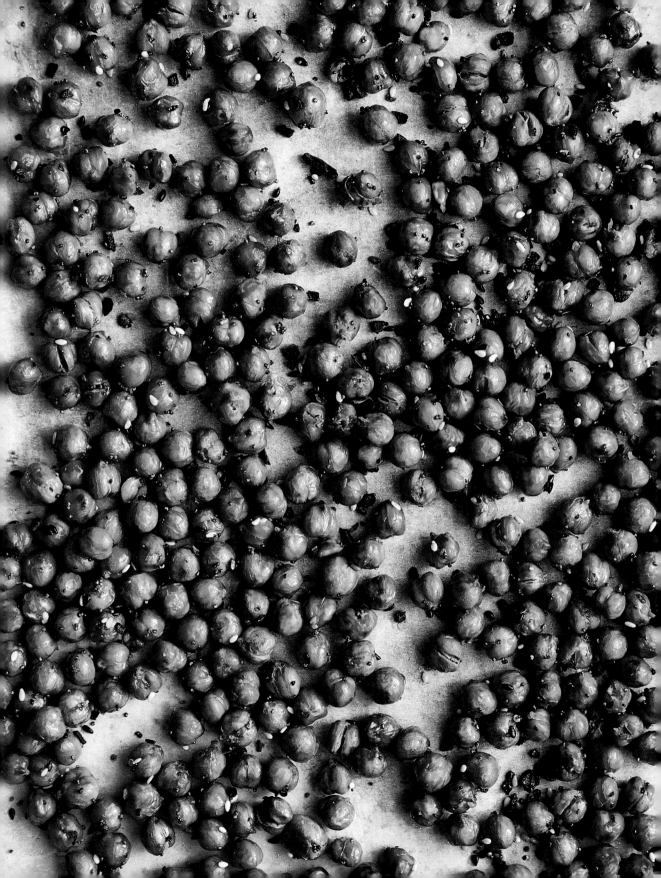

Crispy Roasted "Everything" Chickpeas

These spicy baked chickpeas are quick to prepare and certain to satisfy that craving for a salty, crunchy snack in a nutritious way. For a fraction of the cost of store-bought varieties, you can prepare your own roasted chickpeas and be in control of the amount of added olive oil and salt, choosing seasonings that you enjoy. Seasoned like the famous "everything bagels," these are utterly addictive, and a fiber- and protein-rich snack that you can feel good about eating.

1 (15-ounce) can chickpeas, rinsed and drained

2 teaspoons extra-virgin olive oil

¾ teaspoon sesame seeds

¾ teaspoon poppy seeds

½ teaspoon dried minced onion (see Tips)

½ teaspoon dried minced garlic

¼ teaspoon salt

¼ teaspoon freshly ground black pepper

TIPS: Roasted chickpeas make a great salad topper and nutritious alternative to croutons, and they can also be used as a topping for whole-grain pasta, soups, or vegetables, or folded into a whole-grain wrap for a protein-rich, plant-based sandwich.

Feel free to change the seasonings to your favorites. Or try Indian spices, such as cumin, coriander, cinnamon, and garam masala.

1. Preheat the oven to 400°F. Line a large baking sheet with foil or parchment paper.

2. Blot the chickpeas dry with a paper towel and place them in a small bowl. Add the olive oil, sesame seeds, poppy seeds, minced onion, minced garlic, salt, and pepper. Toss them to coat with the seasonings.

3. Spread on the prepared baking sheet and bake until browned and crunchy, about 30 minutes, watching carefully in the last few minutes of baking to avoid burning.

4. Remove from the oven and allow to cool slightly before enjoying.

5. Store in an airtight container in the refrigerator for up to 1 week.

PER ¼ CUP: Calories: 85; Total fat: 3 g; Saturated fat: <1 g; Cholesterol: 0 mg; Sodium: 100 mg; Potassium: 125 mg; Total carbohydrates: 12 g; Fiber: 3 g; Sugars: 2 g; Protein: 4 g

Lightened-Up Creamed Corn

I grew up with my mom making lots of Pennsylvania Dutch food, a lot of which was doughy, heavy, and made with generous amounts of butter, eggs, and milk. To make her corn pie, first she made creamed corn, which I have lightened up here to retain the signature creaminess of the dish and the seasonings while reducing the excess calories and fat. An extremely nutritious food, corn has a healthy 3 grams of fiber per ½-cup serving and is a good source of vitamin C, magnesium, B vitamins, and the carotenoids lutein and zeaxanthin. Because it is a starchy carb, use this recipe in place of a whole grain as your side along with a green veggie.

4 ears sweet corn, shucked

1 tablespoon coconut oil

1 cup fat-free milk

2 tablespoons all-purpose flour

1 teaspoon sweet paprika

½ teaspoon black pepper

¼ teaspoon salt

TIPS: When you use fresh sweet corn and remove the corn using a box grater or knife, you retain the natural creaminess of the corn, eliminating the need for heavy cream.

If the corn is in season, it should be sweet enough that no sweetener is needed. However, if you like your creamed corn on the sweeter side, simply add a couple of teaspoons of honey or sugar to the recipe. Note that this will change the nutritional count of the recipe.

1. Remove the kernels from the cobs using a box grater (see Tips); you should have about 3 cups.

2. In a medium skillet, heat the coconut oil over medium heat. Once hot, add the corn kernels and cook for 5 minutes, stirring occasionally.

3. In a small bowl, mix together the milk and flour. Add to the corn, stir, and allow to cook until thickened slightly, 10 to 12 minutes.

4. Stir in the paprika, black pepper, and salt. Serve hot.

PER SERVING: Calories: 167; Total fat: 5 g; Saturated fat: 3 g; Cholesterol: 1 mg; Sodium: 189 mg; Potassium: 428 mg; Total carbohydrates: 28 g; Fiber: 3 g; Sugars: 10 g; Protein: 6 g

Quinoa Tabbouleh

Tabbouleh is a traditional Mediterranean grain-based dish made with bulgur wheat, tomatoes, cucumbers, parsley, mint, and lemon. It's full of plant based protein, fiber, and is intensely flavorful. This version swaps the bulgur for quinoa for a slightly different texture and taste, but it retains the signature seasonings of the dish. While not traditional, I like to add some lightly toasted pine nuts for added crunch. A perfect side dish for summer, serve this with hummus or Red Lentil and Roasted Walnut Spread (page 204) and warmed whole-wheat pita bread.

1 cup quinoa, rinsed

Salt

5 tablespoons fresh lemon juice (see Tip)

3 cloves garlic, minced

2 tablespoons extra-virgin olive oil

½ teaspoon freshly ground black pepper

1 tablespoon pine nuts

2 cups finely chopped fresh tomatoes

2 cups minced fresh parsley

1 cup minced fresh mint

2 Persian (mini) cucumbers, diced

TIP: Cooking the quinoa in a bit of lemon juice intensifies the flavor, but you can skip this ingredient if you prefer. If you want to add a bite to the salad, add ½ cup chopped red onion or 2 to 3 chopped scallions.

1. In a medium saucepan, combine the quinoa, 2 cups water, a pinch of salt, and 2 tablespoons of the lemon juice. Bring to a boil, reduce the heat to medium-low, cover, and cook until the quinoa is fluffy but not mushy and the water is absorbed, about 15 minutes. Fluff with a fork and pour into a large salad bowl and allow to cool to room temperature.

2. Meanwhile, in a small bowl, whisk together the garlic, remaining 3 tablespoons lemon juice, the olive oil, ¼ teaspoon salt, and the pepper.

3. In a small dry skillet, toast the pine nuts over medium heat, stirring constantly, until they start to brown, 1 to 2 minutes. Remove from the heat and allow to cool on a plate or in a small bowl.

4. When the quinoa is cool, add the tomatoes, parsley, mint, cucumbers, and pine nuts. Pour in the dressing and mix to thoroughly combine.

5. Serve at room temperature, warmed through or cold.

PER SERVING: Calories: 281; Total fat: 11 g; Saturated fat: 1 g; Cholesterol: 0 mg; Sodium: 203 mg; Potassium: 498 mg; Total carbohydrates: 39 g; Fiber: 7 g; Sugars: 1 g; Protein: 8g

Stuffed Sweet Potatoes with Pistachios and Asparagus

This delicious and super-nourishing sweet potato recipe makes the perfect hearty snack, mini meal, or side dish to go with a light entrée such as grilled fish, chicken, or tofu. Supremely satisfying, the high fiber content of the potatoes and vegetables and the healthy fats from the pistachios keep you feeling full and satisfied. Sweet potatoes are packed with antioxidants including beta-carotene, vitamin C, and vitamin E, and absorption of the antioxidants is aided by the fat in the pistachios, making this an ideal dish for your DASH weight-loss plan.

2 small sweet potatoes (each about 5 inches long), skin well scrubbed

½ cup unsalted pistachios

2 teaspoons grated Parmesan cheese

Juice of ½ lemon

1 teaspoon reduced-sodium tamari or soy sauce

2 teaspoons extra-virgin olive oil

2 cloves garlic, minced

10 ounces asparagus, tough ends trimmed, chopped

2 tablespoons chopped dry-packed sun-dried tomatoes

Salt and freshly ground black pepper (optional)

2 sprigs fresh thyme

1. Prick the sweet potatoes all over with a fork. Place on a microwave-safe plate (see Tip) and microwave on high until very tender, 7 to 12 minutes (depending on the size of the sweet potatoes and the power of your microwave). Remove to 2 plates and let cool for 5 minutes. When cool, split the potatoes lengthwise. Being careful of the steam that will release, open the potatoes wide, and mash the flesh with a fork.

2. In a mini food processor, combine the pistachios, Parmesan, lemon juice, and tamari and process until the mixture is sticky and the pistachios are fine.

3. In a medium skillet, heat the olive oil over medium heat. Add the garlic and cook for 1 minute. Add the asparagus and continue cooking until softened, 3 to 5 minutes.

4. Add the pistachio mixture to the asparagus and combine well. Stir in the sun-dried tomatoes and cook for 2 to 3 minutes to soften the tomatoes. Season with salt and pepper, if desired.

5. Scoop half of the mixture into each sweet potato and garnish with fresh thyme.

TIP: Instead of microwaving the potatoes you can place them on a small baking pan and bake in a preheated 425°F oven for 50 to 60 minutes, until very tender. Let cool for 5 minutes.

PER SERVING: Calories: 409; Total fat: 19 g; Saturated fat: 2 g; Cholesterol: 1 mg; Sodium: 162 mg; Potassium: 1,145 mg; Total carbohydrates: 52 g; Fiber: 10 g; Sugars: 10 g; Protein: 13 g

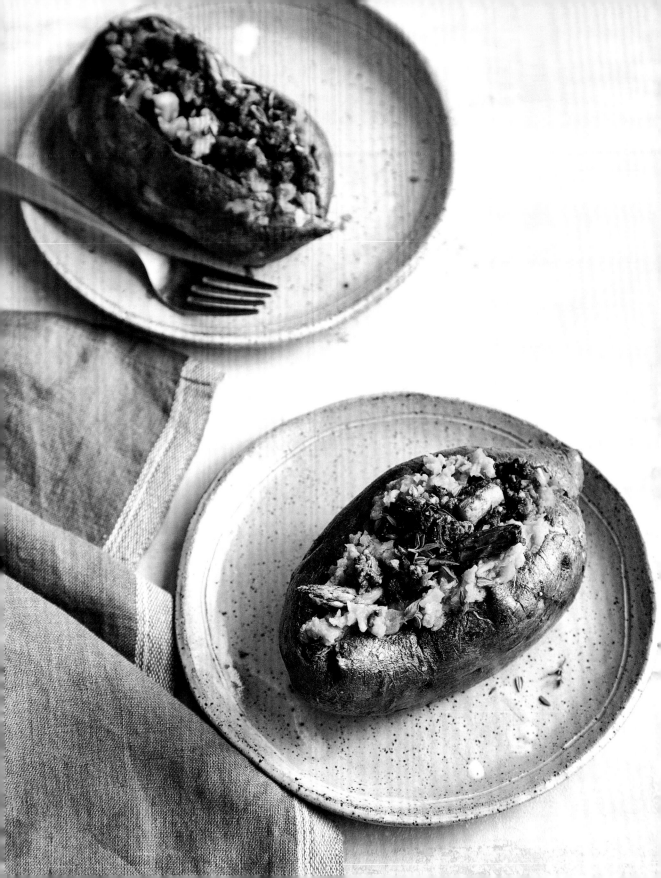

Red Lentil and Vegetable Cakes

These lentil-vegetable cakes are a great way to sneak extra vegetables into your diet. Full of filling plant protein and fiber, lentils lend a nutty, earthy flavor and plenty of essential vitamins and minerals to these tasty veggie cakes. The oats are used as a binder and to add additional cholesterol-lowering fiber. Vegan and gluten-free, enjoy these nutritious patties as a healthy side dish alongside grilled meats or fish. Or have as a snack straight from the oven and serve with Herbed Greek Yogurt Dressing (page 201).

½ cup red lentils, rinsed (see Tip)

1 tablespoon extra-virgin olive oil

½ medium onion, chopped

2 cloves garlic, minced

2 medium carrots, thinly sliced

8 ounces baby spinach (6 to 7 cups)

½ cup rolled oats, plus more as needed

1 teaspoon fresh lemon juice

1 teaspoon ground cumin

1 teaspoon sweet paprika

½ teaspoon dried thyme

¼ teaspoon salt

¼ teaspoon freshly ground black pepper

1. In a medium saucepan, combine the lentils and 1 cup water and bring to a boil. Cover, reduce the heat to medium-low, and simmer until the lentils are tender, about 15 minutes. Drain and transfer to a food processor.

2. In a medium skillet, heat ½ tablespoon of the olive oil over medium-high heat. Add the onion and garlic and cook until slightly golden, 2 to 3 minutes. Add the carrots, cover, and continue cooking until the carrots start to soften, 4 to 5 minutes. Uncover and fold in the spinach and cook until just wilted, 1 to 2 minutes.

3. Preheat the oven to 400°F. Line a large baking sheet with foil or parchment paper.

4. Transfer the contents of the skillet to the food processor along with ¼ cup of the oats, the remaining ½ tablespoon olive oil, the lemon juice, cumin, paprika, thyme, salt, and pepper. Pulse until all of the ingredients are incorporated leaving some texture.

5. Transfer to a large bowl and add the remaining ¼ cup oats. The mixture should be damp but be able to hold its shape. Add more oats if it is too wet.

6. Using a ⅓-cup measure, scoop out portions of the mixture, form into patties, and transfer to the prepared baking sheet. You should get 8 patties.

7. Transfer the patties to the oven and bake until golden brown, 20 to 25 minutes.

8. Remove the patties from the oven and allow to cool before enjoying. They will continue to firm up as they cool.

TIP: Red lentils are used in this recipe because they cook up quickly and aren't as firm as other types of lentils. You can use green or brown if you prefer, but note that the cooking time will be longer.

PER CAKE: Calories: 94; Total fat: 2 g; Saturated fat: <1 g; Cholesterol: 0 mg; Sodium: 105 mg; Potassium: 229 mg; Total carbohydrates: 14 g; Fiber 3 g; Sugars: 2 g; Protein: 5 g

Crispy Baked Zucchini Fries

Although healthy sounding, breaded vegetable appetizers are typically deep-fried and surprisingly high in fat, salt, and calories. This recipe is a healthier alternative, and is a bit of a cross between French fried potatoes and a breaded vegetable appetizer. It's quick to prep and delicious as a side dish or snack. Options are given for vegan and gluten-free, so everyone can enjoy this recipe!

4 medium zucchini (about 1½ pounds)

2 tablespoons flaxseed meal

2 tablespoons grated Parmesan cheese

⅔ cup low-sodium plain whole-wheat panko bread crumbs

1 teaspoon sweet paprika

1 teaspoon garlic powder

1 teaspoon onion powder

¼ teaspoon freshly ground black pepper

1 large egg

2 egg whites

1 tablespoon Dijon mustard

Minced fresh parsley (optional)

TIPS: To make these vegan, use a plant-based milk in place of the egg and substitute nutritional yeast for the Parmesan.

To make these gluten-free, use chickpea panko or another gluten-free panko, or gluten-free oats.

1. Preheat the oven to 400°F. Line a large baking sheet with parchment paper.

2. Cut the ends off of the zucchini and cut into thin spears about ¼ inch wide and 3 inches long.

3. In a shallow dish, combine the flaxseed meal, Parmesan, panko, paprika, garlic powder, onion powder, and pepper.

4. In a small bowl, whisk together the whole egg, egg whites, and mustard.

5. One at a time, dip the zucchini spears in the egg, then dredge in the panko mixture coating all sides of the spears. Place on the baking sheet. Top with any remaining panko mixture. Coat the tops with cooking spray.

6. Transfer to the oven and bake for 15 minutes, then turn and continue baking until browned and crispy, 10 to 15 minutes longer. Serve garnished with fresh parsley, if desired.

PER SERVING: Calories: 116; Total fat: 4 g; Saturated fat: 1 g; Cholesterol: 49 mg; Sodium: 206 mg; Potassium: 565 mg; Total carbohydrates: 14 g; Fiber: 4 g; Sugars: 5 g; Protein: 8 g

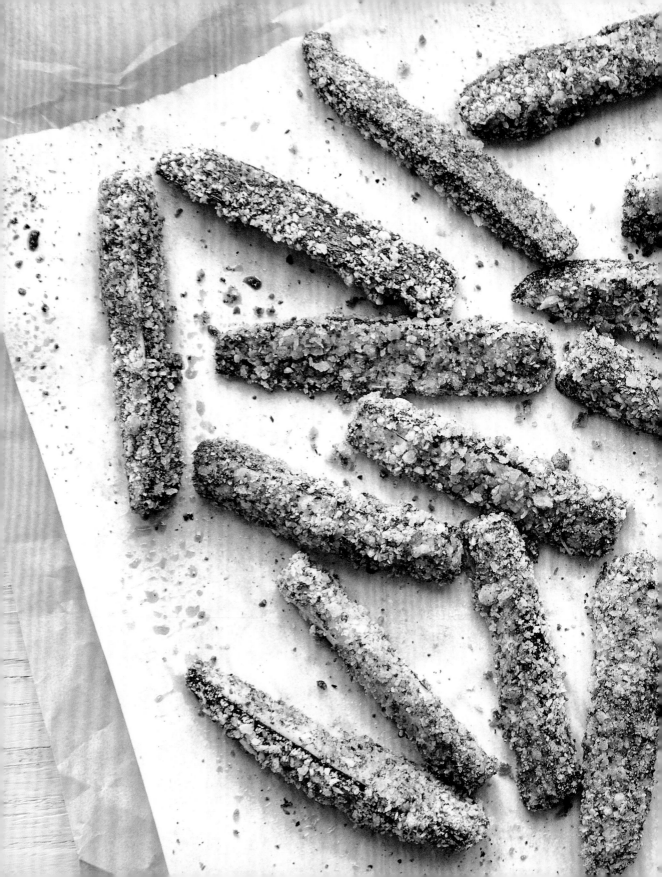

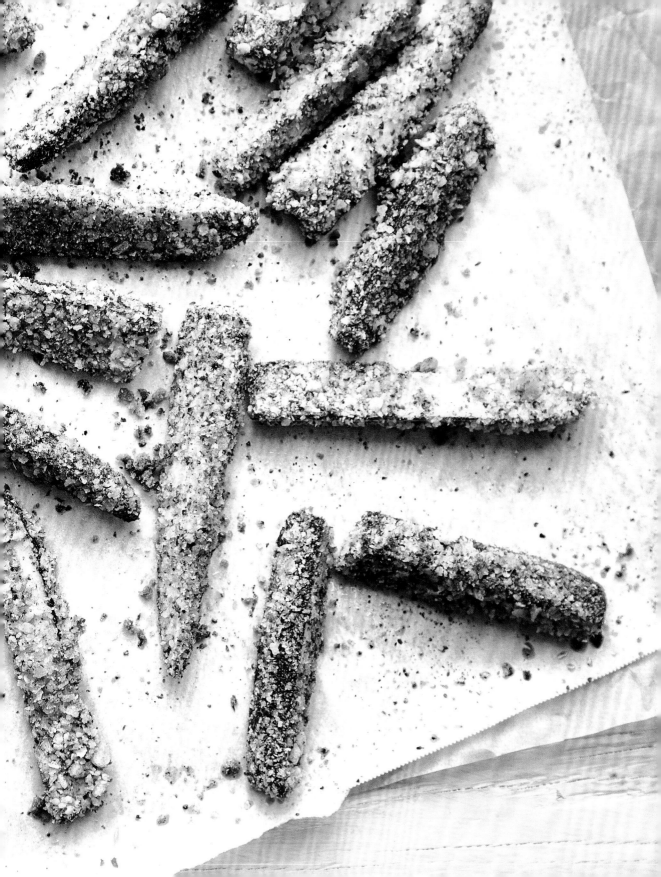

Fall-Spiced Baked Apples

Fruit makes the best dessert, and apples in particular are a good choice when you are managing your weight and keeping your blood pressure in check. High in pectin, a type of fiber that helps to lower cholesterol, apples contain numerous antioxidants and phytonutrients that protect against chronic diseases. A quick-to-prepare and nutritious dessert, apples are topped with slow-digesting fiber-rich oats and a warming mix of spices.

2 large apples

¼ cup rolled oats

2 tablespoons almond meal/flour

2 tablespoons fat-free milk

1 teaspoon coconut oil

1 teaspoon honey

1 teaspoon ground cinnamon

½ teaspoon ground ginger

8 fresh or frozen cranberries

2 teaspoons sliced almonds

1 teaspoon ground nutmeg

TIP: For added protein and to make this a healthy breakfast treat or heartier dessert or snack, top each half with ½ cup nonfat (0%) or low-fat (2%) vanilla Greek yogurt.

1. Preheat the oven to 350°F. Lightly coat a 9 × 9-inch baking dish with cooking spray.

2. Wash the apples and halve through the stem. Carve out the core and seeds with a small paring knife or spoon so that you have a small well in the center. Place the apple halves cut side up in the baking dish.

3. In a small bowl, combine the oats, almond meal/flour, milk, coconut oil, honey, cinnamon, and ginger. Spoon the mixture into the well of each of the 4 apple halves. Top each half with 2 cranberries, ½ teaspoon sliced almonds, and ¼ teaspoon nutmeg. Loosely cover with foil.

4. Transfer to the oven and bake for 30 minutes. Remove from the oven, remove the foil, and pour 1 tablespoon water over each apple. Return to the oven and bake, covered, until fork-tender and slightly browned, for an additional 15 minutes.

5. Serve warm.

PER SERVING: Calories: 135; Total fat: 4 g; Saturated fat: 1 g; Cholesterol: <1 mg; Sodium: 4 mg; Potassium: 156 mg; Total carbohydrates: 25 g; Fiber: 4 g; Sugars: 15 g; Protein: 2 g

Peanut Butter Blondies

As a peanut butter lover, I sometimes indulge a bit too much in this nutritious yet calorie-dense food. Luckily, there's a solution for that, thanks to the brilliant invention of partially defatted peanut butter powder. Readily available in grocery stores, powdered peanut butter has all of the nutrition and far fewer calories than full-fat spreadable peanut butter. With added protein and creaminess from chickpeas without any bean taste, you can indulge in this lightened-up peanut butter blondie recipe without any of the guilt.

1 (15-ounce) can chickpeas, rinsed and drained

½ cup powdered peanut butter

¼ cup rolled oats

¼ cup unsweetened vanilla cashew milk

¼ cup canned unsweetened pumpkin puree

¼ cup granulated no-calorie sweetener (see Tip)

2 tablespoons no-sugar-added creamy peanut butter

2 teaspoons vanilla extract

¾ teaspoon baking powder

⅛ teaspoon baking soda

¼ teaspoon salt

2 tablespoons mini chocolate chips (optional)

TIP: I use granulated stevia for the sweetener in recipes like this to keep calories in check and so I can enjoy a larger portion. However, you could also add ¼ cup honey or maple syrup in its place. Just note that this will change the nutrition numbers.

1. Preheat the oven to 350°F. Lightly coat an 8 × 8-inch baking pan with cooking spray.

2. In a food processor, combine the chickpeas, powdered peanut butter, oats, cashew milk, pumpkin, sweetener, creamy peanut butter, vanilla, baking powder, baking soda, and salt. Pulse a few times to break up the beans, then process until you get a smooth paste, 1 to 2 minutes.

3. Scrape the batter into the pan and smooth out the top with a spatula. If you are using the optional chips, place them on top.

4. Transfer to the oven and bake until a toothpick inserted into the center comes out clean and the top is lightly browned, about 25 minutes.

5. Remove the blondies from the oven and allow to cool in the pan, then cut into 9 squares. Enjoy immediately or store in an airtight container in the refrigerator for up to 1 week.

PER BLONDIE: Calories: 104; Total fat: 3 g; Saturated fat: <1 g; Cholesterol: 0 mg; Sodium: 120 mg; Potassium: 67 mg; Total carbohydrates: 13 g; Fiber: 4 g; Sugars: 2 g; Protein: 6 g

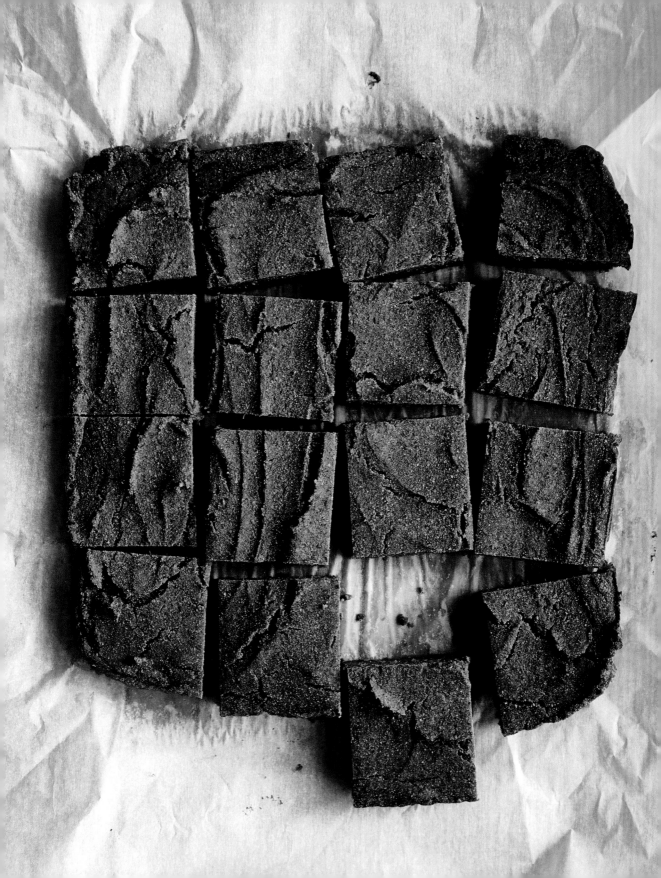

Pumpkin Pie Snack Bars

These pumpkin pie snack bars are made with whole-food ingredients and taste just like pumpkin pie without the crust. Healthier and far cheaper than purchasing processed snack bars, this one-bowl recipe is made without refined sugars and is vegan and gluten-free. Protein- and fiber-rich, and moist like a pumpkin brownie, these are a nutritious and satisfying snack that will keep you feeling fueled.

2 scoops vanilla pea protein powder (see Tips)

1/2 cup coconut flour

1/2 cup granulated no-calorie sweetener (see Tips)

1/3 cup oat flour

1 tablespoon flaxseed meal

2 teaspoons pumpkin pie spice

1/2 teaspoon ground mace

3/4 teaspoon baking soda

1/4 teaspoon salt

3/4 cup fat-free milk

1 (15-ounce) can unsweetened pumpkin puree

TIPS: Pea protein powder is readily available in grocery stores. Extremely versatile, adding pea protein to baked goods is a great way to boost the protein content, the nutrient that keeps us feeling full the longest.

I like using granulated stevia for baking to keep added sugars in check. You can use real sugar if you prefer, just note that this will increase the calorie count.

1. Preheat the oven to 325°F. Line a 9 × 9-inch baking pan with parchment paper.

2. In a large bowl, whisk together the pea protein, coconut flour, sweetener, oat flour, flaxseed meal, pumpkin pie spice, mace, baking soda, and salt. Add the milk and pumpkin puree and mix until completely blended (it will be like a moist dough).

3. Spread into the prepared pan, smoothing the top. Transfer to the oven and bake until the edges begin to brown and the top appears dry, 30 to 35 minutes.

4. Remove from the oven and cool completely in the pan on a wire rack, then refrigerate until cold. Remove from the refrigerator and lift the parchment to remove from the pan. Cut into 16 squares.

PER SQUARE: Calories: 104; Total fat: 2 g; Saturated fat: <1 g; Cholesterol: <1 mg; Sodium: 203 mg; Potassium: 133 mg; Total carbohydrates: 14 g; Fiber: 5 g; Sugars: 3 g; Protein: 8 g

Fudgy Chocolate Black Bean Cookies

Fudgy, chocolaty, moist, and delicious, these quick-to-prepare chocolate cookies get their moistness from creamy fiber- and protein-rich black beans. At just 65 calories per cookie with almost as much protein as an egg, these nutritious cookies can't be beat. Flourless and gluten-free, these healthy cookies make the best guilt-free treat.

4 tablespoons powdered peanut butter

1 (15-ounce) can black beans, rinsed and drained

½ cup unsweetened cocoa powder

½ cup quick oats

¼ cup granulated no-calorie sweetener

¼ cup canned unsweetened pumpkin puree

2 tablespoons fat-free milk

6 tablespoons liquid egg whites (see Tip)

½ tablespoon honey

1 teaspoon vanilla extract

1 teaspoon ground cinnamon

1 teaspoon baking powder

¼ teaspoon salt

TIP: To make this vegan, replace the liquid egg whites with a chia or flax "egg." Mix together 2 tablespoons of either ground chia or flaxseed with 6 tablespoons water and allow to sit for 10 minutes in order to form a gel.

1. Preheat the oven to 350°F. Line a baking sheet with parchment paper or a silicone mat.

2. In a small bowl, stir together the powdered peanut butter and 3 tablespoons water.

3. In a food processor, combine the black beans, reconstituted peanut butter, cocoa, oats, sweetener, pumpkin, milk, liquid egg whites, honey, vanilla, cinnamon, baking powder, and salt and pulse until smooth.

4. Spoon the dough onto the baking sheet, then flatten the tops of the cookies. You should have about 12 cookies.

5. Bake until firm, about 15 minutes. Let cool on a wire rack before enjoying.

PER COOKIE: Calories: 65; Total fat: <1 g; Saturated fat: <1 g; Cholesterol: <1 mg; Sodium: 78 mg; Potassium: 70 mg; Total carbohydrates: 12 g; Fiber: 3 g; Sugars: 2 g; Protein: 5 g

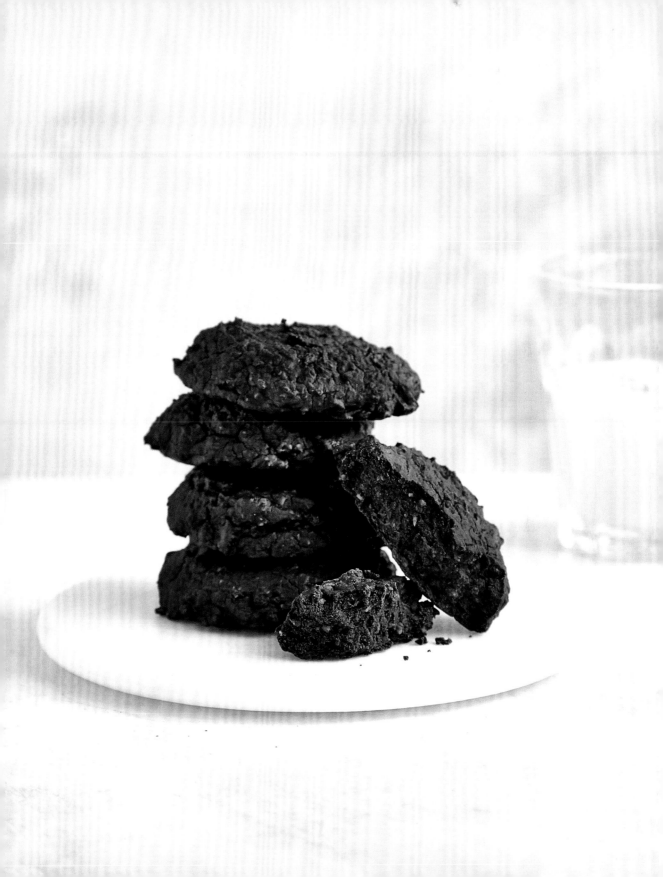

Strawberry-Banana Protein Muffins

Have you heard of "8-a-Day"? It's the California Strawberry Commission's campaign promoting the health benefits of eating 8 strawberries a day. Clinical research suggests that eating just one serving of 8 strawberries a day may improve heart health, help manage diabetes, support brain health, and reduce the risk of some cancers. I created this recipe for my mom a couple of years ago for Mother's Day because she is a huge strawberry fan. So am I. These muffins are sweet, moist, and delicious, and packed with protein, fiber, vitamins, and minerals and certain to disappear fast.

2 ripe medium bananas

1 large egg or 2 egg whites

½ cup nonfat (0%) plain Greek yogurt

¼ cup unsweetened almond milk

2 teaspoons vanilla extract

1¼ cups oat flour

½ cup protein powder (see Tips)

2 tablespoons flaxseed meal

2 teaspoons baking powder

¼ teaspoon ground cinnamon

⅛ teaspoon salt

¼ cup sliced almonds

1 cup diced strawberries

1. Preheat the oven to 350°F. Coat 12 cups of a muffin tin (see Tips) with cooking spray.

2. In a medium bowl, mash the bananas with a fork until smooth. Add the egg, yogurt, almond milk, and vanilla. Mix until smooth and combined.

3. In a separate medium bowl, whisk together the oat flour, protein powder, flax meal, baking powder, cinnamon, salt, and sliced almonds.

4. Add the dry ingredients to the wet and mix just enough to combine. Add the strawberries and stir just to incorporate.

5. Distribute the batter evenly among the 12 muffin cups. Bake until a toothpick inserted in the center of a muffin comes out clean, about 20 minutes. Remove the muffins from the pan and allow them to cool on a wire rack.

TIPS: Plant proteins are generally best for baking as whey protein can make baked goods dry and rubbery. Plain pea protein is a good choice as it has a neutral taste and keeps baked goods moist.

I actually prefer silicone muffin tins because you don't have to spray them and they clean up super fast.

A serving of 8 medium strawberries has a mere 28 calories and provides over 2 grams of fiber, more vitamin C than an orange, and is packed with beneficial antioxidants, phytochemicals, and nutrients, including heart-healthy folate and blood-pressure-regulating potassium. Plus they taste great!

PER MUFFIN: Calories: 120; Total fat: 3 g; Saturated fat: <1 g; Cholesterol: 16 mg; Sodium: 43 mg; Potassium: 277 mg; Total carbohydrates: 16 g; Fiber: 3 g; Sugars: 4 g; Protein: 8 g

Single-Serve Cherry-Vanilla Cupcake

If you have never made a mug cake, get ready for a simple and delicious, perfectly portioned single-serve treat. Mug cakes are made with a short list of ingredients and then cooked in the microwave for less than 5 minutes. Simple to prep with endless variations, this recipe uses nutrient-rich cherries and oat flour with a handful of pantry staples so you can enjoy a healthy sweet treat while losing weight on the DASH diet.

¼ cup oat flour or whole-wheat pastry flour

3 packets (1½ teaspoons) stevia

¼ teaspoon baking powder

Pinch of salt

¼ teaspoon coconut oil

2 tablespoons nonfat (0%) plain Greek yogurt

2 tablespoons fat-free milk

1 large egg white or 2 tablespoons liquid egg whites

½ teaspoon vanilla extract

4 cherries, diced

TIP: You can make this into a confetti vanilla cupcake by adding 1 to 2 teaspoons sprinkles when you mix the dry ingredients.

1. Lightly coat a 10-ounce or larger mug or ramekin with cooking spray.

2. In a small bowl, whisk together the flour, stevia, baking powder, and salt (see Tip). In a separate bowl, whisk together the coconut oil, yogurt, milk, egg white(s), and vanilla. Fold in the cherries. Gradually mix in the dry ingredients until just incorporated.

3. Pour the batter into the prepared mug or ramekin and microwave for 3½ minutes, then check to see if it's set. If needed, add an additional 30 seconds. (Note that because microwaves vary in their power level, always start with the minimum time, then check and continue cooking if necessary.)

4. Immediately run a knife around the edges to help separate the cake from the mug. Firmly place a plate over the mug, flip the mug over, and gently shake the mug to release the cake onto the plate.

5. Let cool for 5 minutes.

PER SERVING: Calories: 180; Total fat: 2 g; Saturated fat: 1 g; Cholesterol: 2 mg; Sodium 237 mg; Potassium: 226 mg; Total carbohydrates: 30 g; Fiber: 5 g; Sugars: 6 g; Protein 11 g

Notes

INTRODUCTION

1. "DASH Eating Plan," U.S. Department of Health and Human Services, National Heart, Lung, and Blood Institute, n.d., https://www.nhlbi.nih.gov/health-topics/dash-eating-plan, accessed June 3, 2018.

HEALTH BENEFITS OF DASH

1. Appel, L. J., et al, "A Clinical Trial of the Effects of Dietary Patterns on Blood Pressure," *New England Journal of Medicine* 336, no. 16 (1997): 1117–24.

2. "High Blood Pressure," American Heart Association, 2018, http://www.heart.org/HEARTORG/Conditions/HighBloodPressure/High-Blood-Pressure-or-Hypertension_UCM_002020_SubHomePage.jsp.

3. Sayer, R. D., "Dietary Approaches to Stop Hypertension Diet Retains Effectiveness to Reduce Blood Pressure when Lean Pork Is Substituted for Chicken and Fish as the Predominant Source of Protein," *American Journal of Clinical Nutrition* 102, no. 2 (2015): 302–8.

4. Whelton, P. K., et al, "ACC/AHA/AAPA/ABC/ACPM/AGS/APhA/ASH/ACPC/NMA/PCNA Guideline for the Prevention, Detection, Evaluation, and Management of High Blood Pressure in Adults: A Report of the American College of Cardiology/American Heart Association Task Force on Clinical Practice Guidelines," *Journal of the American College of Cardiology* 71, no. 19 (2017), https://doi.org/10.1016/j.jacc.2017.11.006.

5. High Blood Pressure. Center for Disease Control and Protection. https://www.cdc.gov/bloodpressure/index.htm.

6. U.S. Department of Health and Human Services, "Physical Activity Guidelines for Americans," 2nd edition, https://health.gov/paguidelines/second-edition/.

7. Champagne, C., et al, "Dietary Intakes Associated with Successful Weight Loss and Maintenance during the Weight Loss Maintenance Trial," *Journal of American Dietetic Association* 111, no. 12 (2011): 1826–35.

8. Blumenthal, J. A. Babyak, M. A., Hinderliter, A., et al, "Effects of the DASH Diet Alone and in Combination with Exercise and Weight Loss on Blood Pressure and Cardiovascular Biomarkers in Men and Women with High Blood Pressure: The ENCORE STUDY," *Arch Intern Med* 170, no.2 (2010): 126–35.

ESSENTIALS OF WEIGHT LOSS

1. Markwald, R. R., et al, "Impact of Insufficient Sleep on Total Daily Energy Expenditure, Food Intake, and Weight Gain," *Proceedings of the National Academy of Sciences* (2013), https://doi.org/10.1073/pnas.1216951110.

2. Foster, J. A., L. Rinaman, J. F. Cryan, "Stress and the Gut-Brain Axis: Regulation by the Microbiome," *Neurobiology of Stress* 7 (2017): 124–36.

3. Seaman, D. R., "Weight Gain as a Consequence of Living a Modern Lifestyle: A Discussion of Barriers to Effective Weight Control and How to Overcome Them," *Journal of Chiropractic Humanities* 20, no. 1 (2013): 27–35.

4. Benedict, C., et al, "Gut Microbiota and Glucometabolic Alteration in Response to Recurrent Partial Sleep Deprivation in Normal-Weight Young Individuals," *Molecular Metabolism* 5, no. 12 (2016): 1175–86.

5. U.S. Department of Health and Human Services, "Physical Activity Guidelines for Americans," 2nd edition, https://health.gov/paguidelines/second-edition/.

6. Neff, K. D., *Self-Compassion: Stop Beating Yourself Up and Leave Insecurity Behind* (New York: William Morrow, 2010).

7. Thompson P. D., et al., "ACSM's New Preparticipation Health Screening Recommendations from ACSM's Guidelines for Exercise Testing and Prescription," 9th edition, *Current Sports Medicine Reports* 12 (2013): 215.

SETTING YOURSELF UP FOR SUCCESS

1. Vartanian, L. R., K. M. Kernan, B. Wansink, "Clutter, Chaos, and Overconsumption: The Role of Mind-Set in Stressful and Chaotic Food Environments," *Environment and Behavior* 49, no. 2 (2017): 215–23.

THE DASH WEIGHT-LOSS MEAL AND EXERCISE PLANS

1. Williams, N., "The Borg Rating of Perceived Exertion (RPE) Scale," *Occupational Medicine* 67, no. 5 (2017): 404–5.

Acknowledgments

I would like to thank my mom and my cousin Bonny Groff for all of their hard work with the bulk of the recipe testing, and all of the eager samplers who gave valuable feedback on the recipes.

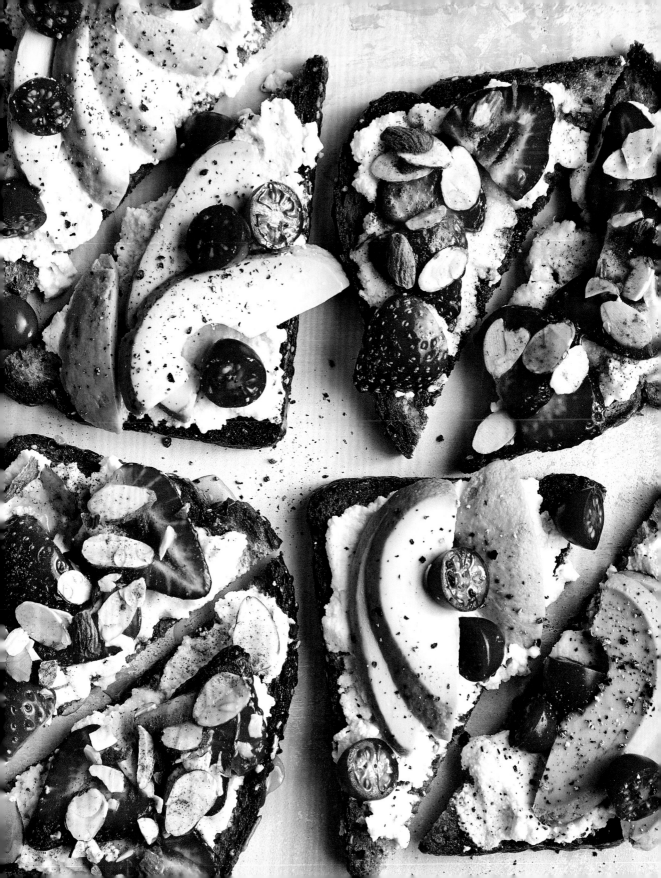

Index

Note: Page references in *italics* indicate photographs.